... Adhering to a program of Pilates, as described in Pilates for Fragile Backs, *under the guidance of a certified instructor can be a most useful means to improve back function and relieve pain. Clearly, this is a valuable therapeutic modality that is underutilized in today's current pain management programs associated with spinal disorders.*

—Charles Birbara, MD, chief of
rheumatology at Worcester City
Hospital in Worcester, MA

In my practice, I constantly emphasize the importance of proper spinal alignment, good posture and a strong mid-section. Pilates for Fragile Backs *highlights these points in an easy-to-follow exercise program for patients suffering with chronic back pain. I have recommended this program to many of my patients, and they are thrilled with the results.*

—Anthony S. Rainka, DC, South
County Chiropractic, Sutton, MA

As a physical therapist, I have been able to utilize the exercises in Pilates for Fragile Backs *with my clients. They have shown a reduction in pain, an improvement in posture and balance, increased strength, and healthier muscle tone. Best of all, the program does wonders for their self-esteem.*

—Pam Craig-Stewart, PT, director of
rehabilitation at Christopher House
in Worcester, MA

This book is a much needed labor of love that offers clear and helpful advice for anyone who has ever lived with chronic back pain. The spine problems addressed in this book are very challenging ones for doctors and therapists alike, and the authors use their firsthand experience with spinal trauma to break new ground for exercise therapy. A specifically modified Pilates program indeed offers the possibility of comfort and relief for a largely under-served group in our society.

—Ellen Kiley, RYT, therapeutic yoga practitioner specializing in scoliosis and spinal fusion

I underwent an anterior/posterior fusion (L4-S1) over a year ago due to degenerative disk disease with annular tears. Since then, Pilates has done wonders for me. I started pursuing basic lumbar stabilization mat work a couple of months following surgery. I had urged my neurosurgeon to allow me to begin sooner than usual because I'd had a big increase in pain. My physical therapist felt it had to do with the stiffness that begins to set in as the weeks go by without stretching and exercising. I had every confidence that Pilates would improve my situation and I swear by it! I've been back to work full-time. I am also walking about four miles, three days a week! I'm sure Pilates for Fragile Backs *will be a major help to many others.*

—Diana Stahl, Cincinnati, OH

Pilates
for Fragile
Backs

RECOVERING STRENGTH & FLEXIBILITY AFTER
SURGERY, INJURY, OR OTHER BACK PROBLEMS

Andra Fischgrund Stanton, LICSW
with Ruth Hiatt-Coblentz

New Harbinger Publications, Inc.

Publisher's Note

Photos on pages 102 and 132 © Peak Pilates.
Photos on pages 103 and 133 STOTT PILATES phototography © Merrithew Corporation.

Distributed in Canada by Raincoast Books

Copyright © 2006 by Andra Fischgrund Stanton and Ruth Hiatt-Coblentz
New Harbinger Publications, Inc.
5674 Shattuck Avenue
Oakland, CA 94609
www.newharbinger.com

Cover design by Amy Shoup; Text design by Michele Waters Kermes;
Cover and Interior Photography by Glenn Harris; Illustrations by Mike Pisiak;
Acquired by Jess O'Brien; Edited by Jessica Beebe

All Rights Reserved. Printed in the United States of America.

Library of Congress Cataloging-in-Publication Data

Stanton, Andra Fischgrund.
  Pilates for fragile backs : recovering strength and flexibility after surgery, injury, or other back problems / Andra Fischgrund Stanton, with Ruth Hiatt-Coblentz.
      p. cm.
  Includes bibliographical references.
  ISBN-13: 978-1-57224-466-5
  ISBN-10: 1-57224-466-6
  1. Pilates method. 2. Back. I. Hiatt-Coblentz, Ruth. II. Title.
RA781.4.S73 2006
613.7'1—dc22
                        2006022230

14 13 12

10 9 8 7 6 5 4

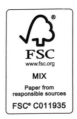
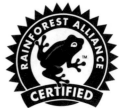

Andra: For Marty, the Cadillac of husbands

Ruth: For Philip and Donald

Contents

Foreword

It is fitting and appropriate to say that the spine is the backbone of the body and must be maintained with care to serve in all the activities of daily living. The spine is called upon in many of the body's functions. As with any machine, improper use, overuse, and inadequate maintenance can cause undue stress and deterioration. When coupled with the natural age-related degenerative changes of the spine, stress and deterioration can lead to pain and even functional disability.

A look at the spinal column demonstrates its complex architecture of bones, muscles, joints, ligaments, and nerves, all intertwined to provide mobility, balance, and protection of the nervous system. A contorted movement by an acrobat will make an onlooker cringe but also marvel at the integrity and flexibility of the healthy spine.

The spine is not made to be stiff or welded together as is done in a spinal fusion operation. However, certain afflictions of the spine—such as degenerative disk disease, trauma, infections, metabolic conditions, and spinal deformities—often require operative interventions. Fortunately, on the other hand, the chronic low back pain that afflicts millions of people from all walks of life can, more often than not, be effectively treated with nonoperative measures.

Pilates body conditioning exercise therapy, which targets the deep postural muscles to achieve core stability, strength, and improved muscle balance, is an appropriate daily routine for any person, and especially those with spinal disorders or deformities both before and after surgery.

Pilates for Fragile Backs is a long overdue book written by an expert in the Pilates method and a patient who has experienced firsthand what it means to regain strength, flexibility, healthy posture, and balance lost through a major spinal fusion operation for scoliosis. This book is a must-read for the able-bodied, for those with chronic back ailments, and for postoperative patients looking for a simple but effective exercise program to reduce pain and restore mobility and function.

As a surgeon treating a multitude of patients with all types of disorders and deformities of the spine, I cannot emphasize enough the importance of proper spine care, particularly for people facing a major spine operation and recovery from such surgery. A Pilates exercise regimen—together with improved techniques in spinal surgery that take into account motion segment preservation, proper alignment, and balance—promises much quicker functional restoration and an easier recovery from spine surgery.

—Oheneba Boachie-Adjei, MD
Chief of the Scoliosis Service
Hospital for Special Surgery, New York

Acknowledgments

Andra warmly thanks model Brigitte Frank for her tireless yet always cheerful participation in this project. She also wishes to thank her surgeon, Dr. Oheneba Boachie-Adjei at the Hospital for Special Surgery in New York; Dr. Karen Bougas at Emerson Hospital in Concord, Massachusetts; the outpatient pool therapy program at Whittier Rehabilitation Hospital in Westboro, Massachusetts; Andrew Southcott of Healing Crossroads Massage Therapy in Concord, Massachusetts; Dr. Vijay Vad of the Hospital for Special Surgery in New York; Cathy Smith of Stott Pilates; Dr. Robert Pashman; and Jess O'Brien of New Harbinger Publications for recognizing the value of this project. Lastly, with all her heart, Andra thanks her Friday Psychotherapy Providers Support Group (Patti, Gail, Leslie, and Ruth), and her husband and her parents for their unfailing love and support.

Ruth wishes to thank Power Pilates of New York City, whose training program and expertise helped make this book possible. She also thanks Dr. Anthony Rainka of South County Chiropractic in Sutton, Massachusetts; Pam Craig-Stewart, physical therapist and director of rehabilitation at Christopher House in Worcester, Massachusetts; and Dr. Richard Tomb. As well, Ruth is grateful to all of her instructors, who continue to guide her in her teaching, and to her clients, who fill her studio with joy. Most of all, she thanks her son, Philip, and husband, Don, whose support enables her own rehabilitation. Their love and patience sustain her each day.

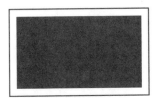

Introduction

Chronic pain is like an internal fire alarm that can't be turned off. It's deafening to you but unheard by others. It can dominate your life so completely that over time, you lose your livelihood and the pleasure of social and family interactions. Your everyday activities and hobbies may no longer seem relevant, and your good spirits and hope for the future drain away. Left unattended, chronic pain can collapse your world into a dark corner of anguish and misery.

We wrote this book to show you that even if you are suffering from chronic back pain as a result of surgical interventions aimed at treating spinal disease, Pilates can safely and effectively ease much of your pain and lead the way to a better quality of life. The exercises are fun and relaxing, too.

It's important that you know you're not alone. Both of us underwent multiple surgeries for spinal conditions and found ourselves relieved of our original sources of pain but facing new ones. Standard physical therapies were temporarily comforting but mostly unhelpful. No one in the medical community seemed to know what additional care to offer besides pain medications, and the side effects of those medications made life difficult in other ways.

The chronic pain addressed in this book can result when the spine is compromised by illness. Sometimes, the surgery employed to treat such illness becomes a cause of pain in itself. Pilates can be helpful for both pre- and postsurgical chronic pain.

In her quest for respite from her suffering, Ruth Hiatt-Coblentz pursued traditional Pilates instruction but modified the exercises, rendering them effective and appropriate for her fragile spine. Once she had mastered them, she introduced them to clients, one of whom was Andra F. Stanton. Andra was so impressed with—and grateful for—the pain relief she experienced using Ruth's regimen, she decided the modified exercises should be put to paper and made accessible to the widest possible audience. Together, Ruth and Andra conceived this book as a gesture of hope and a means to achieve a way out of the cycle of chronic pain. In chapter 1, they'll share their own stories in more detail.

Why Pilates?

Joseph Pilates (1880–1967), a German immigrant, developed his own system of physical therapy based on gymnastics and theories about healthy movement. Originally, Pilates employed his techniques to speed the rehabilitation of his fellow inmates imprisoned during World War I. In the 1920s, when Pilates moved to New York City, professional ballet dancers and athletes turned to him to help repair and strengthen their battered bodies. Many of his five hundred or so techniques gained more widespread popularity in the 1990s when rehabilitation practitioners introduced Pilates methods in orthopedic and geriatric settings as well as chronic pain programs.

Why is Pilates highly recommended for those who have had or may need spinal disk surgery? Unlike aerobic exercises, Pilates uses no quick or jerky motions that often lead to injury. Slow, elegant movements prevail over speed and wasted energy. After a Pilates workout, you generally don't feel exhausted—rather, you feel calm and relaxed.

Though it shares some features with yoga, such as stretching and mindful breathing, Pilates confers less strain on muscles and connective tissues than yoga, especially where fusions begin and end, because it requires less twisting of the torso. Also, Joseph Pilates designed his exercises to be rehabilitative. They're great for the healthy, but they were engineered specifically for the injured. To that end, Pilates—more than yoga or any other exercise regimen—takes into account each individual's physical strengths and limitations and offers a biomechanically complex program of healing.

When you commit to a consistent Pilates regimen, you can expect:

- ◼ stronger muscles

- ◼ a more streamlined shape

- ◼ firmer stomach and buttocks

- ◼ graceful posture

- ◼ improved circulation

- ◼ a decompressed spine

- ◼ lubricated joints

- ◼ an improved sense of well-being

- ◼ pain reduction

All this, without endangering your fragile spine.

The foundation of Pilates is strengthening and stabilizing the core—that is, the trunk muscles—before progressing to peripheral areas. With injured people, the method begins a healing process as a result of increased circulation to injured areas. Joseph Pilates called this improved circulation an "internal shower." His exercise regimens for all—injured and healthy—strive to develop efficient movement patterns that increase strength, balance, and flexibility while building strong muscles.

The core, or trunk, muscles on which Joseph Pilates focused represent the primary muscles responsible for posturally correct and safe movement. They shape the spine into its optimal starting and ending position for all of your activities: bending, reaching, walking, sitting, and so on.

More than three hundred muscles enable your trunk and limbs to move. The strain of faulty movement or poor coordination can eventually lead to spasms, pulls (small ruptures), or tears. And fatigued, strained, or weak muscles cannot follow through with their part in the series of contractions and extensions that make up movement, adding to the potential for injury.

Pilates engages both the superficial or "big" muscles and the deeper muscles, so that entire muscle systems get a balanced workout. Pilates allows overused muscles to begin to disengage, giving them a rest, while weaker, less utilized muscles are strengthened, enabling them to share the stress of movement. For example, among the abdominal muscles, the more superficial muscles (the *rectus abdominis*) and the deeper muscles (the *transversus abdominis* and the *internal* and *external obliques*) form a kind of built-in girdle that supports the torso and stabilizes the spine (see figure 1).

Unlike most exercise programs, which focus on "problem areas," Pilates workouts incorporate movement of the whole person. This "whole person" notion extends to your mind and emotions, as well. That's because Pilates demands intense focus for precision of movement. As a practitioner of Pilates, you must be keenly aware of the positioning of many muscles during any one movement, a requirement that heightens your concentration and your ability to be "in the moment." For this reason, Pilates is never boring.

Further, as you improve the precision of your movement, the ease and beauty of proper motion can offer you a great sense of satisfaction and accomplishment, leading to an improved sense of self-acceptance and positive regard. Pilates, then, is holistic; it creates a mind-body connection.

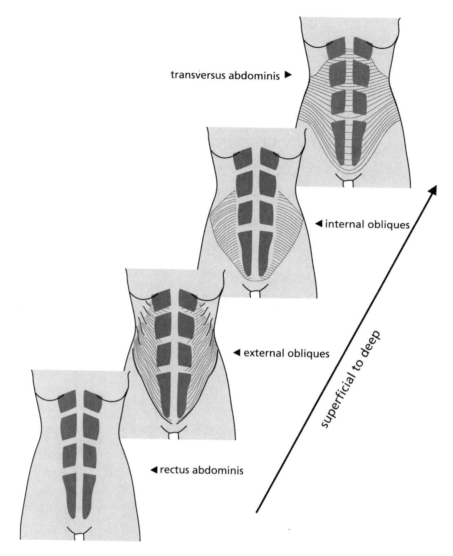

Figure 1: Abdominal Muscles, from Superficial to Deep

Spinal Anatomy: A Quick Review

Let's take a moment to look at the anatomy of the spine so that you can understand how the healthy spine functions and what happens when it is compromised by disease and surgical repair.

To begin, the spine is made up of twenty-four mobile and six nonmobile bones called *vertebrae*. They are stacked on top of each other to form a column. In between each vertebra is a soft, spongy, gelatinous cushion called a *disk*. Each disk is covered by a protective shell. Disks help absorb pressure, like shock absorbers, and keep bone from rubbing up against bone while providing stability to moving parts.

Each vertebra is shaped roughly like a doughnut, so that when stacked on top of each other, the vertebrae form a hollow tube. This tube holds and protects the *spinal cord,* a collection of nerve fibers that carries messages from the brain to the rest of the body. Nerves branch off from two sides of the spinal cord, and each exits through a *foramen,* or space between the vertebrae (see figure 2). Certain conditions can reduce the size of a foramen, and the nerve passing through it can then become compressed.

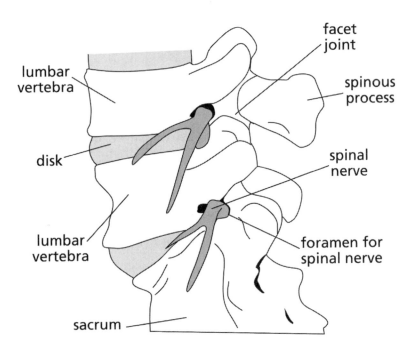

Figure 2: Vertebrae, Disks, and Spinal Nerves

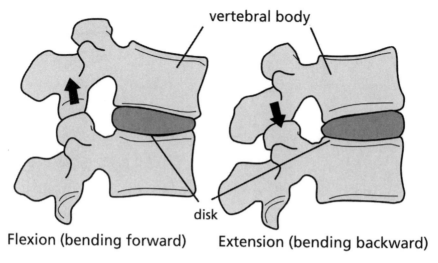

Flexion (bending forward)   Extension (bending backward)

Figure 3: Facet Joints in Motion

Each vertebra has two bony knobs on either side of it that meet the bony knobs of the vertebra above and below it, joining the vertebrae together. The knobs overlap each other to form a *facet joint*. Without facet joints and disks, the spine would not be flexible (see figure 3).

Vertebrae are strapped to one another by soft tissue called *ligaments*. *Tendons* fasten the *paraspinal* muscles—those muscles that lie next to the spine—to the spine. They support the spine and allow the spinal column to move. Smaller muscles control movement between the vertebrae.

The spinal column has four main parts (see figure 4). The *cervical* segment, in the neck, consists of seven vertebrae. The *thoracic* segment, or middle section, consists of twelve vertebrae. The *lumbar* segment, beginning near the navel and ending at the tailbone, comprises five or six vertebrae. Below the spine is the *sacrum* (which contains the coccyx, or tailbone), a group of bones that fuse before birth to form the base for the spine.

All the parts of the spine work together like a well-oiled machine. Collectively, they allow for movement and the body's ability to bear weight. When a part becomes damaged or deteriorates to the point of instability, the spine can no longer function properly.

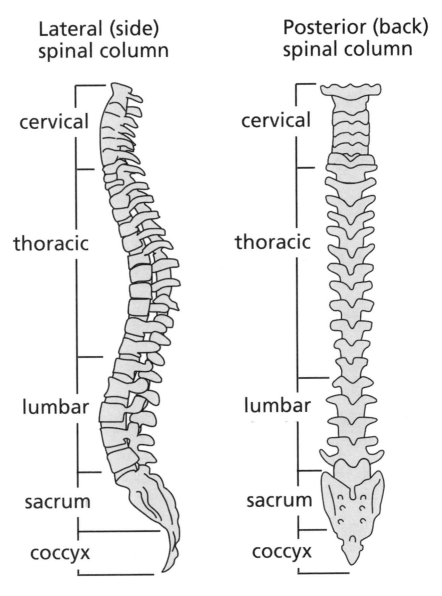

Figure 4: Segments of the Spinal Column

Conditions That Can Cause Pain

Let's take a look at some conditions that often lead to long-term pain.

Herniated, ruptured, or bulging disks. The spinal disk is made of a tough outer layer called the *annulus fibrosis* and a gel-like center called the *nucleus pulposus*. As the spine ages, the nucleus pulposus may gradually lose water content, and a disk's center may be displaced through a crack in the outer layer (see figure 5).

Disk degeneration. Degenerative disk disease is quite variable in its nature and severity. With age, all people will have changes in their disks. Unlike muscles, which have good blood supply, a spinal disk cannot repair itself once it is injured. Without sufficient cushioning, the vertebrae may begin to press against each other, form bony spurs, and pinch a nerve.

Abnormal curvatures. *Scoliosis* is a three-dimensional curvature of the spine, most commonly found in adolescent girls. Scoliosis generally has either a single (C-shaped) curve or a double (S-shaped) curve. Two other types of spinal curvature include *lordosis* (swayback) and *kyphosis* (rounded back). Scoliosis is a sideways curve of the spine,

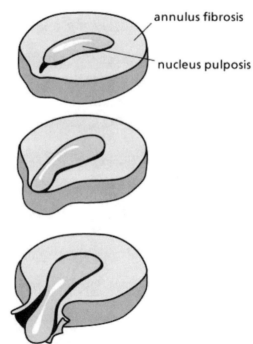

annulus fibrosis

nucleus pulposis

Figure 5: Herniating Disk

lordosis is a forward curve of the spine, and kyphosis is a humplike, backward curve of the spine.

Nerve compression. A herniated disk can press on the nerves in the spine and cause *sciatica,* or pain, numbness, tingling, or weakness in the low back and buttock or down the leg. This process is called *spinal stenosis,* where spinal cord or spinal nerve roots are compressed, or choked. (The term "stenosis" comes from the Greek word meaning "choking.") *Radiculopathy* is pain caused by compression of the roots of the spinal nerves in the lumbar or cervical region of the spine.

Spondylitis. *Spondylitis* is the name given to a group of chronic or long-lasting diseases also called *spondyloarthritis* or *spondyloarthropathy.* These diseases are forms of inflammatory arthritis that primarily affect the spine, although other joints and organs can become involved.

Tumors. Spinal tumors, also called *neoplasms,* are abnormal growths of tissue found inside the spinal column. Such tumors are very rare.

Infections. *Pyogenic vertebral osteomyelitis* is the most commonly encountered form of vertebral infection, although it is considered generally uncommon. It can develop from direct spinal trauma or from the spread of bacteria in the blood to a vertebra. Damage to the vertebrae may lead to kyphosis, which may require surgical correction.

Surgical Treatments That Can Also Cause Pain

Unfortunately, surgical procedures intended to treat back problems can sometimes cause new pain or worsen the original problem. According to government statistics, surgery to relieve pressure on the spinal nerves—including discectomies, microdiscectomies, laminectomies, foraminotomies, and fusions—represent the most commonly performed spinal operations in the United States, with approximately 500,000 taking place each year (Healthcare Cost and Utilization Project 2003). Such surgeries treat disk herniation, disk degeneration, abnormal curvatures, sciatica, spinal stenosis, radiculopathy, and spondylitis, all of which involve compression of the nerve root and cause pain that often radiates to the extremities. The goal of surgery is to decompress the affected nerves.

Surgery should be considered only if significant symptoms persist despite a good trial of nonsurgical treatment. Lucky spinal fusion and disk surgery recipients have little or no long-term back pain. Yet others continue to be besieged by pain years following their surgery. In the worst cases, patients experience *failed back surgery syndrome,* characterized by pain that persists longer than twelve weeks (Wilkinson 1983).

Even among those people who undergo the relatively safe discectomy and microdiscectomy surgeries, as many as 10 percent require second or additional surgical procedures, including fusions, and continued care. Surgery may be less than completely successful due to recurrent disk herniation, stenosis, inadequate decompression of a nerve root, nerve damage, scar tissue formation, or spinal instability.

Apparently, even these fairly simple procedures can create or exacerbate chronic pain (Urban and Roberts 2003).

In fact, of the some 285,000 men and women each year who undergo spinal fusions, up to 40 percent will experience chronic back pain, and as many as 10 percent will actually be worse off than they were prior to surgery in terms of lasting pain (Deyo 2004). A significant number of women and men are destined to find themselves living in a state of debilitation and distress due to fusions intended to cure a chronic illness.

Despite this, over the last ten years or so, the number of spinal procedures performed annually has more than doubled (Herkowitz 1998). A preponderance of back surgery patients say they are never quite the same after surgery. Many back surgeons concede that most patients don't anticipate that surgery often improves the anatomic problems by removing what is pinching the nerve or limiting the blood flow, but it does not return the patient to a predisease condition.

Because about 26 million visits are made to physicians' offices every year due to back pain, and because back pain is the second most common medical complaint in the country (American Academy of Orthopaedic Surgeons 2000), it seems clear that chronic back pain and sometimes the surgical procedures used to treat it present a widespread and significant public health challenge.

If your surgery was suggested and performed by an experienced, knowledgeable, and conservative physician, chances are you needed your spinal surgery. But even the best surgeons will tell you only if pressed that many back surgery patients return to them with complaints of enduring pain. Few patients facing spinal surgery understand that the goal of being pain free following surgery is very often unattainable.

Spinal Surgeries

Surgical strategies to repair spines have changed over the decades as understanding of the biomechanics of the spine improves and as better instrumentation and techniques are developed and become available. Since there are many possible permutations of vertebral damage, each patient's individual situation will influence the decision about the appropriate kind of surgery.

Microdiscectomy

The current standard procedure for lumbar disk herniation is a *microdiscectomy*. The surgeon begins by making a two-inch incision in the lower back. With the aid of a surgical microscope, he pushes aside the skin and soft tissues, exposing the bones of the spine. The surgeon then uses a retractor to spread apart the bones of the vertebra, makes a slit to expose the nerve root, and lifts the root so that he can get a good view of the damaged disk.

The surgeon slices open the tough shell of the disk and scoops out the nucleus. If the nerve root is still being compressed, he may consider enlarging the foramen or removing the *lamina,* a bony projection off the back of the vertebra. Finally, the surgeon puts the muscles and soft tissues back in place and stitches the skin together. Many patients leave the hospital a day after surgery.

Spinal Fusion

If, however, spinal instability results from complications of previous surgical procedures, a fusion may be deemed necessary to ensure the integrity of the spinal column. Surgeons also recommend fusions when a patient has an abnormal curvature, such as scoliosis or lordosis, that is likely to get progressively worse. *Spinal fusion* entails welding together a group or groups of vertebrae so that the bones heal into a single, solid bone.

Patients can undergo a *posterior fusion* (with the incision made in the back), an *anterior fusion* (with the incision made in the abdominal area), or both. In all cases, the spine is repositioned into the best alignment that can be achieved and then held in place with metal *instrumentation*—rods, hooks, wires, and screws. Natural or manufactured bone chips are positioned between the vertebrae, sometimes in cages, and the bone chips grow together, resulting in a fusion. It takes a year or two for the bones to fuse completely.

Once they fuse together, segments of the spine—especially in the lumbar region—lose their normal range of motion. (Figure 6 illustrates the normal range of motion.) A lumbar fusion limits sideways bending as well as the ability to bend backward and, to a lesser extent, forward. Moreover, nonfused segments take on the full load of movement, subjecting them to massive wear, or *junctional degeneration*. The fewer vertebrae removed from action, the more likely it is that junctional problems in adjacent vertebrae will result. The more extensive the fusion, the more movement will be restricted.

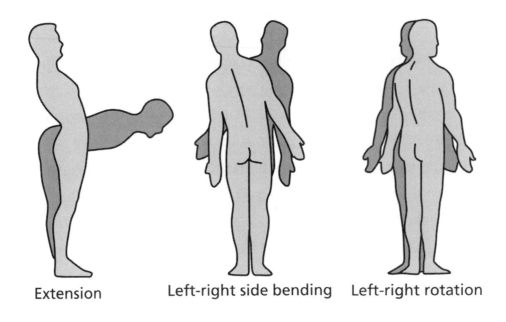

Extension   Left-right side bending   Left-right rotation

Figure 6: Normal Range of Motion

How to Use This Book

Before you begin any exercise program, you absolutely must obtain consent from the surgeon who performed or will perform your spinal fusion or other surgical procedure. It is our understanding that most people should wait a full year following surgery before undertaking a strenuous exercise program, because it can take a year or more for fusing bones to completely join together. Until then, warm-water pool therapy, gentle walking, basic stretching, the recumbent bicycle, and the elliptical machine pose the least danger to your healing spine.

Because Pilates exercises target each person's particular needs, we also stress that when you decide to begin this workout program, you should find a certified instructor in your community and work closely with that person for a while. In this way, you will be sure to learn correct positioning and the essential techniques that are the foundation for all Pilates work. Also, your instructor will have the opportunity to confirm that the exercises suggested in this book are appropriate for you.

We highly recommend that you bring this book to your instructor so that she can follow the regimen Ruth adapted for sensitive spines. Your instructor might even further modify your routine in light of any special needs you may have. An added advantage to working at first with an instructor lies in the verbal cues she will use to remind you how to organize your torso and regulate your breathing. You will find that you will repeat these cues to yourself as you do the workouts on your own.

After your first few sessions, you might feel very sore—but a good sore, the kind that comes from warmed-up, stretched-out muscles. If you feel pain, however, you should let your instructor know immediately and stop your sessions if necessary.

If you find yourself feeling extremely tired after many of your first sessions, don't let it deter you. Take care of yourself—rest, sleep, relax, soothe your sore muscles—and go to your next session and practice, practice, practice.

General Dos and Don'ts for Pilates Workouts

◼ Do obtain permission from your surgeon or health care provider before beginning these exercises.

◼ Do stop if you experience pain, shortness of breath, faintness, dizziness, palpitations, or a rapid pulse when resting.

◼ Do work on a slip-resistant mat.

◼ Do tie up long hair.

◼ Do wear comfortable clothing (similar to yoga attire).

◼ Don't wear shoes; bare feet will help you avoid slipping.

◼ Do be sure to drink plenty of water throughout and after your workout.

◼ Do remember that with Pilates, less is more. You're aiming for quality, as opposed to quantity, of movement.

◼ Don't exercise just after eating a large meal.

◼ Don't ever change exercises midstream. Completely finish one before beginning another.

◼ Don't exercise if you've taken medication that makes you sleepy or makes you unaware of your pain.

◼ Do practice two to three times weekly—or more often.

Everyone's Different:
Our Stories

In this chapter, we'll look at two common paths to spinal fusion surgery. Advanced or rapidly progressing scoliosis, or curvature of the spine, represents the most common medical condition that necessarily leads to spinal fusion surgery.

Andra will share her experience with scoliosis and spinal fusion. Disk disease and injury also can lead to a fusion, depending upon the type and severity of vertebral breakdown and the judgment of the attending surgeon. Ruth will share her story, which followed this path.

Scoliosis

Scoliosis is characterized by one or more abnormal side-to-side spinal curves, often in the shape of an **S**, an **L**, or a **C**. Frequently, these curves can cause the spine to rotate like a spiral, potentially constricting the heart and lungs and compromising their functioning (see figure 7). Present in 2 percent to 4 percent of children between the ages of ten and sixteen, scoliosis is a relatively common condition. Scoliosis affects primarily preadolescent and adolescent girls, who are five times more likely than boys to have a rapidly progressing form that requires medical intervention. The average curve progresses about one degree per

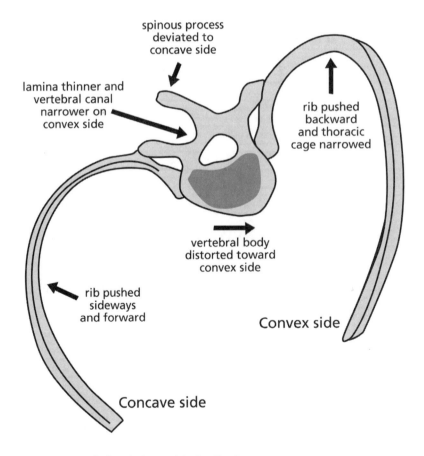

Figure 7: Rotation of the Spine with Scoliosis

year, and curvatures of over fifty degrees almost always call for spinal surgery (Neuwirth 1996).

Scoliosis is an *idiopathic* disease, meaning that the cause remains unknown. However, children of parents with scoliosis have a 20 percent greater likelihood of developing the illness than children with no such family history (Neuwirth 1996). Therefore, a genetic (hereditary) component seems to underlie this disease.

Children are now routinely tested for scoliosis in school. Warning signs of the onset or development of scoliosis in children and young adults include:

- ▣   One shoulder is higher than the other.

- ▣   The head is not centered directly above the pelvis.

- ▣   One hip is higher than the other.

- ▣   The two sides of the rib cage are at different heights.

- ▣   The waist is uneven.

- ▣   The trunk is leaning to one side.

- ▣   One side of the back is higher than the other when bending over.

This is Andra's story. Stricken with scoliosis at the age of eleven, she has spent the rest of her life managing pain symptoms associated with this disease and the two surgical procedures that both helped and harmed her.

◘ Andra's Story

My mother first noticed my spine wasn't straight when she saw me in a bathing suit at the beach. I was eleven years old. She took me to three local orthopedic specialists on Long Island, New York, who took X-rays and confirmed that I had an L-curve. Each physician told my mother there was nothing that could be done, and so my disease progressed until my spine had twisted in a spiral and my left-side ribs had migrated to my back. One leg was shorter, one hip bone was higher, and I had developed a hump.

When I was eighteen, while my sister was waiting to be interviewed for nursing school, she picked up a newsletter in the waiting room of Columbia-Presbyterian Hospital in Manhattan. When her name was called, she stuffed the newsletter in her purse. At home, my mom found it and read an article about how orthopedic surgeons were performing spinal fusions for those with progressive scoliosis.

As you would guess, a short time afterward, in the late 1970s, I had my first spinal fusion. My fifty-six-degree curve was corrected to twenty-five degrees, and I had a Harrington rod installed for stabilization while my bones fused. I was sent home in a twenty-five-pound plaster body cast that started at the groin and ended at my chin. In back, it continued upward to form a headrest. I wore it for nine months—with no showering. I was eighteen and forever traumatized. To have had my body exposed to so many medical and hospital personnel and to be seen in such an ugly contraption, especially as an adolescent, was mortifying. I hibernated most of those nine months, while all my friends went off and experienced their first year of college.

I had minor pain now and then over the years, but for the most part, I was able to do all the things I needed to do. Still, I was always concerned about damaging my fusion, and so I avoided activities that carried a higher than average risk of sending me flying, falling, or twisting, which meant that I steered clear of nearly all athletic activities.

Then, about twenty-five years after my surgery, I started to develop back pain. A rheumatologist prescribed a muscle relaxer (Flexeril, or cyclobenzaprine) and daily walking on a treadmill or outside. At first, I was so stiff that I could barely stretch my legs enough to walk without pain. With time, the medication relaxed my muscles and they stopped irritating the nerves that were signaling pain to my brain. I was finally able to walk—and eventually even jog.

When I developed *bursitis* (inflammation of the sac between the tendon and the bone) in my hips, three years later, I could no longer walk for exercise. Cortisone injections helped in the short run, and lots of Ultram (tramadol, a non-narcotic painkiller) combined with Tylenol (acetaminophen) kept me going for a while. Ultimately, though, I developed unbearable sciatica in one leg and referred pain in my other ankle that felt like a fracture that would not heal. I sought out surgeons because I knew I would need more surgery—it had just been a matter of time.

What was going on—and what goes on for nearly every scoliosis patient who had a spinal fusion before 1990—was that I was experiencing pinched nerves due to a narrowing of the spinal canal and the foramina (holes) that let the main nerve root branch off into the body's extremities. This was partly because the bones in my spine never fused properly, or perhaps the fusion broke early on; either way, my vertebrae continued to shift, meeting at unnatural angles and rubbing up against one another.

In addition, I was developing *flat back syndrome,* a problem caused by my original surgery. The surgeon had reshaped my spine to be straight from side to side, but this plan did not take into account the spine's natural, mild front-to-back curves. These curves help to balance the loads carried by the spine. So my spine had been molded into another abnormal shape. This is what all scoliosis surgeons were doing at the time. They didn't know it would turn out to be a problem in years to come.

My goals for the second surgery were to relieve the pinched nerves and flat back syndrome, and to fuse the spine to prevent the vertebrae from shifting around again. In terms of these goals, the surgery was a success. I was thrilled to be rid of sciatica and referred pain. As part of my recovery, I took part in warm-water therapy, to regain balance and help restore lost muscle tone and strength, and later added "land" therapy that included stretching and using the recumbent bicycle and a fitness ball.

Yet unexpectedly, I found I had a new source of pain—my upper back. It wasn't difficult to understand what was going on. Now that my lumbar spine was finally fused and immobilized, the stress of all of my movement fell on the part of my back that still could move: the part above my new fusion. That, in turn, exacerbated the *osteoarthritis* (degeneration of the joints) that had developed where my first fusion met up with my natural spine. After years of bearing the brunt of much of my movement, my upper back finally was falling apart, too.

My surgeon was sympathetic and referred me to physical therapy. After several trials of physical therapy, however, I still had chronic pain between my shoulder blades and in the tops of my shoulders and my neck.

The drawback of most physical therapy, it seems to me in retrospect, is that it is both too passive and too conservative. My last physical therapy trial, comprising twice-weekly visits over eight weeks, involved ultrasound, electrical stimulation, heat packs, and mild massage. I was also sent home with basic stretching exercises to do as often as I could tolerate. It felt great to have my sore back massaged and heated, but soon after I left the physical therapist's office, my pain returned.

Because I was under the misconception that I should avoid exercise after a fusion and certainly when I was in pain, and because this idea seemed to be supported by the relatively passive treatment I was receiving, I was afraid to pursue exercise. I knew for certain, for example, that I shouldn't take part in a lot of jumping, so that ruled out aerobics. I knew it was impossible (and perhaps even dangerous) for me to arch and twist, so that ruled out yoga and Pilates—at least it ruled out the positions that practitioners typically use on their book and DVD covers to represent those modalities. What was left?

By this time, I was taking medication for depression. If you've ever had pain, you know how lonely an experience it can be. To look at me, you would have thought I was doing okay, and in many ways I was. I could go food shopping, vacuum a little, and cook. But I couldn't hold down a paid job anymore. I sometimes found myself crying if I was seated in the car too long (more than fifteen minutes), for instance, or if I needed to run more than one errand a day, since that often started what I call a "pain process," a series of worsening symptoms that—unless treated with bed rest, heat, and medication—mushrooms into a prolonged bout of pain and downtime. Since no one could see an external manifestation of my pain, it seemed to me like my unhappy secret.

And I found it confusing. As people age, most everyone experiences pain. So how could I claim to be in more pain than the next aging person? Was it okay to acknowledge my pain, to take it seriously—or was it better to deny it, minimize it, and rise above it as best I could? To own up to it seemed to me like malingering (wanting attention), and as a psychotherapist, I knew this was a shameful diagnosis. Yikes! My feelings ran the gamut of self-doubt, guilt, self-reproach, sadness, helplessness, hopelessness, and depression. It took a long time to finally give myself permission to have chronic pain—that is, to recognize and acknowledge that it has played a big part in my life.

I now understand, too, that exercise and movement are essential in my bag of tricks for managing back pain. Prolonged inactivity actually increases my pain, because my back becomes stiff, weak, and out of condition. By pursuing modified Pilates, I have made my spine more flexible and strong. I now have days when I'm pain free, though I'm not every day. Still, it's a significant improvement. I feel more in control, too, and psychologically empowered. If I'm hurting, I know what to do to find some relief. I'm so happy I found my Pilates instructor, Ruth. I trusted her with my broken body because hers had been broken as well.

Disk Breakdown

For most people who sustain a serious back injury, the injury is not an isolated incident. Rather, over the years, accumulated stress from misuse and overuse add up, causing a slow degeneration of the spinal disks, which weakens the back and renders it vulnerable to harm.

Degenerative disk disease is a result of accrued wear and tear on the vertebrae. In the worst instances, the inner, gelatinous center of the cushions, or disks, between the bony vertebrae dry out and shrink, narrowing the openings through which nerves run, pinching those nerves, and leading to back and leg pain and leg weakness.

Nearly everyone over forty has some degeneration of the lumbar disks. This is a natural result of age and use. By the age of fifty, approximately 85 percent of Americans will show signs of disk breakdown. Some of these people experience pain, and the more fortunate do not. The diagnosis of degenerative disk disease is given to those who experience low back pain three months or longer (Gunzburg, Szpalski, and Andersson 2004).

Although degeneration of the disks is a gradual process, certain activities—such as lifting, twisting, and bending—tend to increase the stress on damaged disks. As the degeneration progresses, the disk loses its ability to act as a shock absorber, and vertebrae can collapse on one another.

For mild cases of disk degeneration, treatment often entails brief bed rest followed by a relatively quick return to physical activity. The temptation—and the prescription by physicians—to limit activity can actually exacerbate the condition. Physical therapy (ultrasound, heat, and massage) and exercise to strengthen the back and abdominal muscles, when tolerated, offers the best route to recovery.

More severe cases that do not respond to traditional physical therapy or exercise call for more intensive treatment. For example, if spinal stenosis (narrowing of the foramina) develops, a *laminectomy* (a surgical procedure in which the *lamina,* or roof, of a spinal vertebra is removed in order to enlarge the vertebral openings) might be unavoidable. In the most severe circumstances of degenerative disk disease, spinal fusion becomes necessary. A fusion restores adequate space through which the nerves may pass and ensures the longevity of this reconstruction.

There is a movement afoot to avoid spinal fusion altogether for people with degenerative disk disease who have not developed stenosis and sciatica. Nonfusion technologies, such as artificial disks, represent a different kind of surgery to resolve the problem of damaged disks and the pain they cause. In 2004, the United States Food and Drug Administration approved the first such disk, made of plastic and metal and implanted between the vertebrae, replacing failing natural disks. Early studies suggest that disk replacement reduces pain and allows for a quicker recovery, greater spinal flexibility, and less stress on adjacent structures than fusions (Zeegers 1999). But without long-term studies, it remains unclear whether this procedure will prove more helpful than the more traditional fusion.

Moreover, some people with disk deterioration and without nerve compression might not require surgery of any kind. For example, a recent Swedish study indicated that though a fusion decreased pain over the first years following surgery, no differences in the long run were reported by those who had fusions and those who did not. After five to ten years, all study participants described approximately the same levels of pain (Anderson et al. 2003).

The best solution to early stage disk disease may very well be a strenuous but safe exercise routine coupled with a serious commitment to ongoing spinal care, which might include medication, massage therapy, ice or heat, and emotional support. Beginning such a program sooner rather than later can help prevent the formation of adhesions and unnecessary scar tissue, and increase the blood supply to devitalized muscles surrounding the spine, thereby providing enhanced circulation essential for healing.

> *Ruth's story involves disk degeneration coupled with spinal injuries. After accidents and years of strenuous exercise routines resulted in the collapse of several vertebrae, Ruth underwent surgery with a physician whose skills were out of date. As a result of all of these circumstances, she has spent most of her adult life in debilitating pain.*

◻ Ruth's Story

As a teenager, I was in a minor car accident and, a short while later, probably dislocated a disk while lifting a heavy pan of dishes. From that point on, my back seemed to become susceptible to injury.

The next injury of serious consequence occurred when I was twenty-one; a chair was pulled out from under me, and I went crashing to the ground. I was hospitalized briefly and sent home with instructions to stay in bed.

Over the years, whenever my back caused me discomfort, I was treated with cortisone injections and bed rest. But neither of these interventions proved very helpful, so I decided to try something different. I began to engage in high-impact aerobic exercises and weight training. Looking back, the aerobics probably put extra pressure on my spine, but I always felt so much better after exercising.

I followed this strategy over the next twenty years or so. But in my forties I was in a serious car accident, and a few years later my car was rear-ended while I was at a stoplight. After these accidents, I began to notice that I was in pain more frequently than ever before and that this state of affairs was affecting my ability to go about my usual activities. For example, I had trouble driving back and forth to my graduate school classes—and sitting through them, as well.

On one particular day, after standing for an extended period at school and then driving home, I started out for a walk. Along the way I heard something snap in my back, and I knew immediately that something was very wrong. I felt sure I would need surgery.

I sought out only one opinion, from a surgeon at a large teaching hospital near my home. I made the mistake of limiting my choices to local surgeons when I should have gone to a major city to look for an expert physician in a hospital, center, or program that specialized in fusions. Scans revealed that the disk between my bottommost vertebra (lumbar vertebra number five) and sacrum had completely degenerated, as had the disk between the first and second lumbar vertebrae.

> If you've been told you're a candidate for spinal fusion, you should search out the most widely respected surgeons who specialize in spinal fusions before undergoing surgery. Even better, get two or three opinions, if possible. Don't settle for the surgeon or facility that's most convenient.

Although I called for an appointment in September, I was not given one until January, at the teaching hospital in town. I should have seen that as a red flag. Hospitals that are knee-deep in red tape cannot efficiently accommodate their patients. In contrast, large medical facilities in big cities—despite their size—generally manage to avoid long delays in scheduling appointments for serious conditions.

Ultimately, I underwent eight hours of surgery. I was never given pain medication afterward. I was in extraordinary pain, and in the end it was for nothing, because my surgeon had used an outdated procedure; he had used wire around the fusion site instead of a rod and pedicle screw system.

Four months after the first procedure, my back started to spasm, and I could barely walk. My surgeon would not see me. He referred me to his physician's assistant and ordered prescriptions for pain medication. I sought out a second surgeon, who ordered a discogram, a procedure that revealed which of my spinal disks had deteriorated. But that second surgeon was reluctant to perform the extensive revision surgery I needed, and he never returned my phone calls to discuss the results of my tests and a date for surgery, so I moved on.

I finally turned to a spine surgeon at a well-known Boston hospital. I knew I had found the right doctor. He explained to me that my first fusion had caused the collapse of my lumbar spine. He urged me to undergo a second fusion and insisted on meeting my family to prepare them for my postoperative recovery. Of course I agreed to the surgery.

Soon after my surgery, I felt well enough to return to a gym and engage in mild to moderately strenuous exercise, including something new: Pilates. In fact, I found that Pilates was the one type of exercise I could always do, no matter how bad I felt, and it would never fail to bring about improvement.

Pilates has served me in two major ways: psychologically and physically. After spinal surgery, my confidence was diminished when it became painfully obvious that my body no longer functioned as it once did. I thought that I might never be able to work again. After studying and practicing Pilates, however, I found that my mobility and spinal flexibility were much improved. Though my life has taken a different direction and my surgery has been the end of one lifestyle, Pilates was the beginning of another one for me.

After I had spinal surgery, my muscles lost their flexibility. My balance was thrown off due to the fact that my hip alignment had changed and my body weight was distributed differently. Often, through lack of strength, I tended to hinge forward, particularly when fatigued. However, because Pilates emphasizes the lengthening and strengthening of muscles associated with the spine, and enhances balance through proper alignment, I was able to re-educate my body. Once again I am able to perform daily chores that include simple tasks such as bending and lifting.

I continue to experience pain, though the degree depends on many factors, such as the weather, how many hours I've worked, and fatigue. But Pilates has limited the intensity and frequency of my pain so that I never have to turn to pain medication. When I feel that my body needs realignment, I simply get on my equipment and work out until the pain dies down. Pilates has become my analgesic.

I continue to take lessons every week, and I have learned from experienced instructors how to restructure various movements to suit my limitations. As well, I have learned from personal experience that when some part of an exercise feels uncomfortable, I will be able to find my own modifications. I approach that part in a slightly different way, without changing the goal of the exercise, and I almost always come to a point where I can complete the entire exercise.

This combination of learning from other instructors and creating, on my own, something that is appropriate for my medical condition has guided me in creating the modifications that I now share with my clients. Since there are so many different roads to an end result in Pilates, I never feel cheated or inadequate. I find that the more I teach, the more I learn, so that this process never becomes tedious. It has been an enriching experience and continues to be so.

2

Taking Care of Body, Mind, & Spirit

If you have had surgery for back disease or injury, or if you are suffering with back disease or injury, it is imperative that you take extra special care of yourself. Pursuing Pilates at least twice a week is a must, even though taking on another major commitment in your busy life may seem daunting if not impossible. It *is* possible, and you need to make it happen. If you don't, you will end up paying for it in the long run in the form of spasms, burning, and other kinds of discomfort—or, worse, a decline in your ability to do the things you need and want to do in your life.

The wonder of the human body is that it is tough and resilient, but it is also fragile at the same time. Amazingly, we recover from all sorts of physical insults and injuries: sprains, fractures, cuts, bruises, and surgery. Yet we rarely get away from injury without repercussions. Because the body is so complicated and its interconnected systems so delicate, nudging the system off course is bound to have consequences. Frequently, by compensating for something that has gone awry, our bodies operate under duress.

It's important to attend to your body, your mind, and your spirit. Some of what you can do for yourself is effortful, but other measures don't require much effort at all. The easiest changes to make involve simply buying—and using—products and services that support and soothe the back, and avoiding situations that can lead to or worsen pain symptoms. The point is that living with a fragile back calls for making some lifestyle changes. By making these changes, you will most certainly decrease the stress and strain on your already compromised bones and muscles. Here are our suggestions.

Basic Body Mechanics

Some of the simplest changes you can make involve the way you support your back during your everyday activities: sitting, standing, sleeping, lifting, and carrying.

Support While Seated

Most people slouch when seated for a long period. This posture strains the lower and upper back. When fitted and placed correctly, a support pillow will help you avoid slouching by keeping your ears, shoulders, and hips in alignment while maintaining the normal inward curve of the lower spine. Overall, a lumbar support keeps the spine in a neutral, natural position.

Although many lumbar support pillows and rolls are portable, your best bet is to purchase one for every chair you use daily and leave them all in place. For example, have one for your home office chair, your desk chair at work, your reading chair, your chair at the kitchen table, and your relaxing chair, and have one for your car as well.

Make sure your lumbar supports don't push your lower back forward too far. If they do, try a softer model, or try another manufacturer's product line. We suggest experimenting with samples from specialty stores that have an easy return policy. What feels right in the showroom might not suit you when you actually use it at home or at work. Likewise, you might find that what provides comfort in your reading chair irritates you in your car. For that reason, you probably will need a few different kinds of support pillows, and there is really no way to discern what will work in a showroom. See Resources for retailers that sell lumbar supports.

If you have an extensive lumbar fusion, a lumbar support may not be necessary, since you have built-in support in the form of metal rods and bolts. In fact, a support placed higher on the chair might be more helpful for you. Held in place with an elastic belt, such a support adjusts easily, keeping the thoracic and cervical spine nice and straight, and prevents slouching, which can inflame nerves in the neck and shoulders.

IMPORTANT TIPS FOR SITTING
AT YOUR COMPUTER

To avoid neck discomfort while working at your computer, place the monitor directly in front of you, not angled to one side or the other, at about one arm's length away. Adjust the monitor height so that the top of the screen is just below eye level. This will ensure that your neck stays in a neutral position (angled no more than fifteen degrees downward).

Never hunch forward while working at a desk or table. Also, rather than sitting in an erect position (with your hip joint forming a ninety-degree angle), try to recline slightly (aiming for a one-hundred-ten-degree angle instead).

A footrest can relieve pressure on the lower spine while you work at your desk. A phone book, sturdy box, or other stable object will do the job. Position the footrest so that your knees are level with your hip joint, and place your feet flat on the footrest.

Support While Sleeping

You spend about a third of your life sleeping, so it makes sense to take some time to choose the sleep system that best suits you. What should you look for in a mattress? Everyone is different, but generally, a mattress designed to conform to the spine's natural (or engineered) curves will keep the spine in alignment. It will distribute pressure evenly across the body and allow for good circulation and a comfortable night's sleep.

Above all, don't keep a sagging mattress. If necessary, place a board under it or put it on the floor until you can make better arrangements. Likewise, when you shop for a replacement, don't buy a mattress that allows you to sink into it. On the other hand, a mattress that is too firm will put pressure on those parts of your body that have the most contact with it—the hips, sacrum, shoulders, and head—leading to pain and stiffness. You might want to consider a mattress that allows you to vary its firmness (see Resources). Again, you will need to try out several mattress systems in store showrooms. Choose stores with a free return guarantee of at least thirty days.

Similarly, look for pillows designed to keep the spine in natural alignment. Experiment with different heights, degrees of firmness, and shapes. Down pillows generally provide the least support, while down-and-feather pillows are firmer but still provide the fluffy feel of a down pillow, if that's what you're after. Some people swear by latex or contour-foam pillows, and others like the malleability of buckwheat-filled pillows.

To enhance any pillow, you might try using a cervical roll. Slip it inside the pillowcase with your pillow or position it on top of the pillow so that it rests right up against the inward curve of your neck. This setup provides support to the neck without pushing the shoulders forward and stressing the spine.

Sleeping on your side with your knees slightly bent promotes back health, especially if you use an extra pillow between your knees to relieve stress on the hips. If you sleep on your back, a firm pillow beneath your knees will take some pressure off your spine. Try to avoid sleeping on your stomach, because this position really strains the neck. If you can't resist, consider using an oversized body pillow up to your collarbones and resting your forehead on a roll or other small pillow so that you avoid twisting your neck.

Support While Standing

Just as when sitting, when people stand, they tend to slouch. When you slouch, your head is thrust forward, the upper spine is overly rounded, the pelvis tilts forward, and your knees lock, all leading to back problems.

In contrast, ideal posture keeps your body weight evenly distributed on the skeletal frame, minimizing wear and tear on bones and muscles and providing vital organs with the room they need to function normally. To achieve ideal posture, visualize a plumb line hanging down from each earlobe. The plumb line should drop straight down through the shoulder, down the middle of the arm, and through the anklebone. The chin should be pulled in slightly and the shoulder blades pulled down and slightly back, keeping the chest open but not pushed forward. The pelvis should shift slightly forward, allowing the hips to align with the ankles.

Lifting

Use posture that protects your spine whenever you need to lift objects—and try to avoid lifting heavy objects. To pick up an object that is lower than waist level, don't bend forward at the waist. Instead, squat down by keeping your back straight and bending at your knees and hips. Stand completely upright without twisting, and move your feet forward as you lift the object.

If lifting an object from a table, slide it to the edge of the table. Bend your knees, and use your legs to lift the object as you come to a standing position. Hold the package close to your body and keep your stomach muscles tight. To lower the object, tighten the stomach muscles and bend at the hips and knees.

Carrying

If you use a handbag, tote, briefcase, or laptop computer case, try to carry only items that you really need. Otherwise, you risk applying too much force to one side of the body, causing or exacerbating neck, shoulder, or back strain.

Backpacks tend to cause less strain, but only if you use both shoulder straps. Don't sling a backpack over one shoulder. The shoulder straps should be wide, padded, and adjustable. Using a hip strap along with the shoulder straps is even better. A loaded backpack should not exceed 15 percent of the body's weight and should never weigh more than twenty-five pounds. When loading your pack, position heavier items close to your back. Finally, consider using a wheeled backpack and, ideally, push it rather than pull it.

Soothing Sore Muscles

After you exercise, your muscles may feel tired and achy from stretching. Your muscles may also cramp, spasm, or burn due to overuse, incorrect use, inadequate use, or injury. You don't have to—and shouldn't have to—live with pain. Here are some of the many options available to you for soothing sore muscles.

Hot Baths and Heating Pads

Superficial heat in the form of *hydrotherapy* (hot baths) and heating pads is helpful in diminishing pain and decreasing local muscle spasms. Hot baths and heating pads are especially good for providing comfort when muscles are sore and achy from an active exercise program.

A study published in the journal *Spine* reported that heat was significantly more effective than either ibuprofen or acetaminophen at reducing muscle stiffness and pain, leading to greater flexibility in patients with acute lower back pain (Nadler et al. 2002).

Hydrotherapy with bath salt formulas represents an ancient treatment for muscle and joint pain. A recent study at the University of Birmingham in the United Kingdom confirmed that both blood magnesium and sulfate concentrations increased after Epsom salts baths, although the amount of absorption varied from person to person, with men showing slightly higher levels of blood magnesium than women and women showing higher levels of free plasma sulfate than men. Magnesium is said to be a natural muscle relaxant and anti-inflammatory, and sulfate breaks down toxins and removes them from the body (Ahsan 1997).

Warm Epsom salts baths perfumed with an essential oil such as lavender or peppermint can help relax both the body and the mind. Simply fill your tub with the warmest water you can comfortably tolerate, pour in two cups of Epsom salts, add aromatherapy ingredients if desired, and soak for fifteen to twenty minutes, adding hot water if necessary to keep the bath warm.

Transcutaneous Electrical Nerve Stimulator Therapy

A *transcutaneous electrical nerve stimulator* (TENS) machine is a small, battery-operated, portable device that delivers electrical current through electrodes attached to the skin, using very small doses of electricity to generate heat in targeted nerves. Theoretically, the heat relieves stiffness and pain by stimulating the body's production of *endorphins,* brain chemicals that serve as natural painkillers and produce feelings of well-being.

You will need a prescription to purchase a TENS unit, and you should consult with a physician to make sure you don't have a condition (such as having a pacemaker) that contraindicates TENS therapy. Though pricey versions are routinely used by physical therapists, inexpensive brands (from $80 to $100) can be obtained over the Internet (see Resources). The cheaper models offer fewer options but can be effective, if you find TENS helpful. You may also find it useful to consult with a physical therapist to learn how to use your unit.

TENS machines were first introduced more than thirty years ago as an alternative to medications for chronic pain, but their usefulness remains clinically unproven. In a 2002 article in the journal *Spine,* for example, Brosseau and colleagues found no difference between subjects who received electrical stimulation from a TENS unit and those receiving stimulation from a dummy unit. Yet for many, twenty or thirty minutes of TENS can feel as good as a massage, and they swear by it.

Warm-Water Pool Therapy

If your insurance policy covers it and you don't have a condition that contraindicates it (such as having a pacemaker), we highly recommend warm-water physical therapy (not water aerobics) as one of the first exercise regimens to use following spine surgery. The water should be ninety degrees or warmer. This therapy improves balance, stretches muscles, relieves pressure on the spine, begins to strengthen the muscles that support the back, and can be very soothing physically and emotionally.

Moving in deep water causes a mild traction effect on the spine. This occurs because two opposing forces are at work: the compressive force of gravity and the buoyant effect of water. The traction effect can be increased by the use of ankle weights, along with a flotation belt or tube at chest level. Gravity pulls the feet downward while the flotation device maintains the position of the upper body. Traction decreases pressure between vertebral disks and may increase foramen size. Blood flow and oxygen delivery are significantly increased during immersion, as is the removal of muscle metabolic waste products.

Massage Therapy

Many ancient peoples—including the Greeks, Egyptians, and Chinese—were convinced of the therapeutic properties of massage and used it to treat a variety of ailments. These days, massage is thought to increase circulation and reduce inflammation. Deep tissue massage, in fact, may be one of the most effective nonpharmaceutical treatments for inflammation. Massage can also increase the elasticity of ligaments and muscles, and it has a general relaxing effect on the body.

Surprisingly, few studies of massage for back pain have been undertaken, considering the popularity of massage. Those that have been conducted, however, have shown positive results. For example, in a small Canadian study, participants with low back pain who received a comprehensive program involving stretching, massage, exercise, and soft tissue manipulation reported less disability and pain than those performing exercise alone (Preyde 2000). In another, larger study, researchers randomized patients with chronic low back pain to receive either acupuncture, massage, or educational materials. At the conclusion of the study, the subjects who received massage showed better functioning than those receiving acupuncture or self-care educational materials (Cherkin et al. 2001).

Generally, although a single massage will probably be helpful for you, the effects of massage are cumulative, so a course of massage treatments will likely bring about the greatest benefits. Regular massage can have the effect of reducing painful spasms and areas of muscle tightness, strengthening and toning the entire body, and helping to prevent strains and injuries that might otherwise occur, especially when there is already structural damage or weakness. And one of the nicest benefits of massage is a feeling of deep calm, thought to be caused by the release of endorphins.

Because many different forms of massage exist, it can be confusing to choose the type that is most appropriate for your needs. A brief description of some of the most popular types of massage may be helpful.

SWEDISH MASSAGE

A popular and ubiquitous form, *Swedish massage* is a vigorous style designed to energize the skin and nervous system and stretch ligaments and muscles, maintaining or restoring suppleness in these areas. The therapist uses rolling, kneading, and percussive strokes to manipulate and relax the soft tissues. Swedish massage purports to shorten recovery time from muscular strain by flushing the tissue of lactic acid and other metabolic wastes.

Swedish massage may in fact be too vigorous for people with spinal fusions and degenerative disk disease. If you pursue this form of massage, be sure to inform the massage therapist of your surgery, existing instrumentation or artificial disks, and other areas of tenderness from surgery or illness.

TRIGGER POINT, SHIATSU, AND DEEP TISSUE MASSAGE

Trigger points are tight, spasming muscles or painful, palpable knots that sometimes feel like a pinched nerve. Trigger point, shiatsu, and deep tissue massage aim to alleviate muscle spasms and cramping. The therapist palpates, locates, and deactivates painful areas where muscles have been damaged or developed a reoccurring spasm. Pressure is briefly applied to these trigger points, which can be momentarily painful but ultimately greatly relieving. The muscles are then gently stretched to complete the relaxation process.

This massage style endeavors to reduce spasms by releasing muscle tissues that have become stuck to one another and inducing new blood flow into the affected areas. Spasms are partly maintained by a nervous system feedback cycle in which pain causes a spasm which in turn causes more pain. Since spasms reduce blood flow to the trigger point, which reduces oxygen supply to the tissues and increases the spasm, activating blood flow through massage likely stops the cycle.

CRANIOSACRAL THERAPY AND MYOFASCIAL RELEASE MASSAGE

Craniosacral therapy and *myofascial release massage* represent much gentler forms of massage. They are an alternative to the more physically forceful Swedish and trigger point techniques. Both are becoming increasingly popular for a wide range of medical problems associated with pain and dysfunction.

With these methods, the recipient lies on a massage table fully clothed. The practitioner applies very slight pressure—no more than the weight of a nickel. Therefore, spinal fusion recipients and those with degenerative disk disease don't risk unintentional irritation of or damage to soft or deep tissue.

Every muscle is covered by a *fascia,* a thin layer of tissue. Like a stocking, the fascia holds all internal structures in place, helps maintain body posture, and provides support and strength to the muscles. But the fascia can tighten or become stuck together in places, constricting muscles and preventing them from fully relaxing. The craniosacral therapy practitioner gently stretches the fascia along the direction of the muscle until the tissue releases and fully elongates. As a result, posture improves and cramped muscle groups relax.

SELF-MASSAGE

Here is a simple self-massage technique you can use to help relieve muscle pain. Securely tape two tennis balls together with duct or shipping tape. Then, place the balls on your mattress and very slowly lie back onto them. If you don't go especially slowly, you're likely to bruise yourself, so be cautious. Your goal is to position yourself so that the massager is gently pressing against the spasming muscle.

Once you are lying on the double-ball massager, you may find it needs to be placed elsewhere against your back to get at the right spot. So sit up, move the massager around, and each time you move it, lean onto it very carefully. Once you hit the right spot, you'll know it immediately because your pain will disappear. It might not work for you every time, but when you're in pain, it's worth giving it a try.

Pain Control

Pain was once believed to be a person's cross to bear. Unless in the throes of a fatal illness, patients were expected to tough it out. Fortunately, those sentiments no longer hold sway, and chronic pain is now considered a disease state all its own. In this section, we'll discuss some approaches to pain control.

Botox Injections

The FDA has approved the use of Botox (botulinum toxin) for pain relief, and clinical trials have confirmed the efficacy of this treatment for some back pain (Foster et al. 2001). Derived from the same substance that causes botulism, Botox is modified for medical use and injected into the paraspinal muscles of the neck or low back to relax spasms. The substance works by temporarily paralyzing these muscles.

Gradual relaxation of the back muscles occurs over a week or two and can last for two or three months or longer. Injections are administered in a physician's office or under sedation in an outpatient medical care facility. Temporary side effects may include a brief increase in pain and soreness at the site of the injections. It is not yet clear whether positive effects continue to be achieved with repeated injections.

Cortisone Injections

Cortisone is a hormone naturally produced by the adrenal gland above the kidney. When a semiartificial form is used as an injection, it becomes a useful tool to suppress inflammation, dissolve scar tissue, and promote healing.

The effectiveness of cortisone injections is not a sure thing; sometimes the injections work, and sometimes they don't. If cortisone does work, its pain relief can last up to six months. However, there is a limit to how many times you can get these injections. This is partially due to the fact that after a while, cortisone may start breaking down healthy tissue once damaged tissue has been eradicated.

Cortisone injections fall into three categories: trigger point injections, facet joint injections, and epidural injections.

CORTISONE INJECTIONS TO
THE TRIGGER POINTS

Cortisone injected into trigger points relaxes the muscle so that blood flows into the area, washing out irritants and promoting healing. Some trigger points require multiple injections. This treatment may leave you feeling bruised and sore for a short while.

CORTISONE INJECTIONS TO THE FACET JOINTS

These injections are directed at the facet joints, or spaces between vertebrae as they stack up on each other and form the vertebral spinal column. Facet joints allow the spine to bend forward and backward and to twist. Cortisone injections reduce inflammation in the facet joints, breaking the pain cycle and making it possible to begin physical therapy.

EPIDURAL CORTISONE INJECTIONS

Epidural cortisone injections affect the space just outside the protective covering of the spinal cord. Filled with blood vessels, this space surrounds the *dura* membrane that holds the spinal nerve roots and the fluid that bathes the roots. With disk herniation, for example, these areas can become inflamed.

Epidural injections not only deliver pain-relieving medication directly to the inflamed tissues, but they are also said to flush away inflammatory proteins that contribute to future pain, thus breaking the pain cycle for several months.

Chiropractic

Scientific literature supports the efficacy of chiropractic treatment of lower back pain. However, when seeking chiropractic care, choose a licensed, credentialed practitioner who offers nonforce or low-force techniques and has extensive experience with disk conditions and spinal fusions. Stay away from those who use forceful manual adjustment techniques, since these may further damage a fragile spine.

During an acute phase of pain, a chiropractor employs standard orthopedic and neurological testing to determine the type and location of the spinal problem. A postural analysis, investigation of spinal joint motion restrictions, and measurement of pelvic balance might also be used to ascertain a diagnosis.

Once the diagnosis has been reached, the practitioner then stretches, or tractions, the spine. Gentle pumping eventually forces the disk to return to its proper position, shifting it away from the nerve it is impinging upon, reducing inflammation and associated pain.

Pain Medication

A variety of pain medications are available to help alleviate pre- or postsurgical back pain.

NONSTEROIDAL ANTI-INFLAMMATORIES

Most physicians and pain specialists commonly recommend an over-the-counter *nonsteroidal anti-inflammatory* such as ibuprofen (Advil, Motrin) or naproxen (Aleve). These aim to decrease muscle inflammation, which may in turn decrease nerve stimulation. Some prescription anti-inflammatory medications, *COX-2 inhibitors* such as Celebrex (celecoxib), are considered unsafe due to cardiovascular complications arising from their use.

MUSCLE RELAXANTS

Muscle relaxants constitute a group of drugs that have a sedating effect on the entire body, including the muscles. Flexeril is the only one that has been deemed safe to use on a long-term basis, because it is not habit forming. It can be very effective at relieving spasms, stiffness, tenderness, and pain, but many people find it overly sedating. By taking it in gradually increasing doses, though, some eventually get used to this medication and use it successfully.

Other muscle relaxants, such as Soma (carisoprodol) and Valium (diazepam), do become habit forming and are therefore typically prescribed on a short-term or as-needed basis. They also can be quite sedating.

NEURONTIN

Another non–habit forming medication that may offer help to pain sufferers—especially those with nerve pain—is the antiseizure medication Neurontin. Its effectiveness as a pain reliever has not been well studied and scientifically proved, and anecdotal reports vary widely.

TRICYCLIC ANTIDEPRESSANTS

In low doses, a tricyclic antidepressant such as Elavil (amitriptyline) appears to diminish pain, though the mechanism for this action is not known. Tricyclics also relieve sleep problems because of a powerfully sedating side effect. A problem with this type of medication is that with higher doses, its side effects (including dry mouth and constipation) become intolerable for most.

ULTRAM

Ultram, a relatively new entry to the market, has no anti-inflammatory effect but acts centrally on the brain, like nonsteroidal anti-inflammatory medications, to modulate the sensation of pain. It may be a good option because it is not addictive with extended use and can be quite effective if well tolerated.

OPIOIDS

Finally, narcotic or opioid pain medications also help manage pain, but they are strong and potentially addictive. Therefore, physicians consider them only if nothing else proves helpful. Commonly prescribed narcotics include Tylenol 3 (acetaminophen with codeine), Vicodin (hydrocodone), and Percocet (oxycodone).

Opioids act by attaching to receptors in the brain, spinal cord, and gastrointestinal tract. As with other medications that act on the brain, they effectively change the way a person perceives pain. Some people muse that opioids don't relieve pain; instead, they make you forget about it. Indeed, narcotic medications affect regions of the brain associated with pleasure, resulting in the euphoria described by many who take them.

Long-term use can lead to physical dependence, but some doctors contend that people with chronic, debilitating pain should nevertheless be prescribed opioids. If taken correctly, these medications allow people to become more functional. They may be enabled, for instance, to reenter the workforce, enjoy activities with friends and family, and have a psychologically empowering sense of better control over their pain levels.

Physicians agree that discontinuation of opioid use should always be medically supervised in order to avoid or alleviate withdrawal symptoms. These symptoms can include restlessness, muscle and bone pain, fever and chills, insomnia, gastrointestinal distress, and involuntary muscle movements.

All medications, even over-the-counter analgesics like aspirin and acetaminophen, have the potential for side effects. No medication is perfect. Your use of medication should be overseen by a physician or comparable caregiver. Ideally, medication should not be relied upon as the sole source of pain reduction and relief.

MORPHINE PAIN PUMP

For those people with intractable pain who cannot find relief through more conservative therapies, an intrathecal drug delivery system, more commonly known as an implanted morphine pump, represents a last resort.

According to the medical device maker, Medtronic, over 50,000 individuals throughout the world rely on a pump system to treat severe, chronic pain or spasticity. In fact, intrathecal drug delivery systems have been in use since the 1980s.

In 1997, the most advanced pain pump, the SynchroMed System, developed by Medtronic, received approval from the US Food and Drug Administration. The size of a silver dollar, this pump is implanted in a subcutaneous pocket of the abdomen and connected by catheters (thin tubes) to the spine. The unit lasts from five to seven years after which it needs to be replaced.

When a dose of medicine is administered, the pump places medicine directly into the cerebrospinal fluid that surrounds the spinal cord. As a result, the medication doesn't have to circulate through the body before reaching the pain-sensing areas of the brain. The effect is immediate, only small doses are needed, and there are fewer or less potent side effects than with medicines taken by mouth.

The pump is usually programmed to deliver doses continually. The unit needs to be refilled regularly, so the patient needs to work closely with a pain management program.

Managing Depression

People with enduring pain often develop emotional disturbances, especially clinical depression. Symptoms of depression include:

- sad mood

- decreased motivation to do the things you normally do

- apathy (lack of interest in hobbies, friends, or family)

- irritability

- feelings of worthlessness or guilt

- poor concentration

- impaired ability to sleep

- an increase or decrease in appetite

- anxiety

- impaired memory

- decrease in sexual desire

- ▣ fatigue

- ▣ thoughts of death

If you have five or more of these symptoms, and they are persistent, you may be experiencing severe depression. Women in particular tend to develop additional complicating problems such as anxiety, weight gain or loss, and oversleeping.

Emotional stress brought on by pain tends to heighten sympathetic nervous system activity, which may further amplify the perception of pain. This forms a continuous loop of pain leading to depression and depression leading to a heightened awareness of pain. For this reason, people with clinical depression should strongly consider trying ongoing antidepressant medication therapy. If you are clinically depressed, these medications can give you the motivation and psychological energy you need to begin an exercise regimen and pursue other methods of pain reduction and control as well as psycholgical comfort.

Once you have mustered the motivation to seek help for depression, finding an antidepressant medication that reduces your symptoms without intolerable side effects can be a frustrating experience. Several trials, each taking a week or so, are often required. Some unlucky people may never find a satisfactory solution. Still, it's definitely worth experimenting since many people do respond well and experience few or no side effects.

The newest classes of antidepressant medications, *selective serotonin reuptake inhibitors* (SSRIs), and a combination of an SSRI and a *norepinephrine reuptake inhibitor* (SSNRI) are vast improvements over older medications. Unfortunately, though, SSRIs and SSNRIs can have their own unpleasant side effects. Even the blockbuster drug Prozac (fluoxetine) works for just over half of the people who try it. Nonetheless, antidepressant medications can be very useful for people living with chronic pain.

Isn't it ironic that when a person is feeling severely depressed, with little energy or motivation and an inability to think clearly, she must begin the sometimes arduous search for an acceptable antidepressant? Many people give up the search, and that's understandable. But it's very important to stick with the process. It will be necessary to work closely with someone who is knowledgeable about the most recent pharmacological treatment for depression—a primary care physician, physician assistant, internist, psychiatrist, or, in some US states, a nurse with an advanced nursing degree. Find someone you like and trust to accompany you on your mission.

Support Groups and Psychotherapy

In most communities, through hospital outpatient clinics, mental health clinics, or community programs, you may come across support groups for those with chronic illness. Even if you are not a joiner or a talker by nature, attending a support group can be very helpful—first and foremost because it shows you that you are not alone with your pain. As group members discuss their own predicaments, you may begin to feel that others can relate to what you experience with your own chronic pain, and this can be tremendously comforting.

Spinal fusions or degenerating disks aren't obvious; no one can see them. Many fusion recipients and disk breakdown sufferers choose not to divulge their "secret." Since our culture places such a high premium on good health, few want to expose the fact that they have a medical condition and therefore risk being thought of as abnormal. So most suffer in silence, feeling isolated and estranged from coworkers, friends, and family.

Using the Internet to enter forums and chat rooms specifically for fusion recipients and those with disk injury or disease can be quite helpful, but forming compassionate relationships with others in the real world will probably prove to be even more enriching and satisfying, although it takes more courage.

Of course, if you want support but get panicky—or turned off—just thinking about joining a group, by all means find a psychotherapist, preferably one with a current or past chronic illness of her own, and make a commitment to that relationship for several months. Psychotherapy frequently helps to get your feelings off your chest, offers a witness to your life's troubles, and helps you find out if issues from your past make it particularly difficult for you to accept or cope with your situation. Most importantly, psychotherapy can help you discover how to resolve those issues.

If you find yourself feeling and thinking in very negative, self-defeating ways, a psychotherapist who specializes in cognitive behavioral therapy can teach you specific techniques that will get you to think more positively about your life. This can be particularly helpful in coping with chronic pain.

Mind Over Matter

As sufferers of back pain, we both doubted that techniques like self-hypnosis, meditation, or progressive muscle relaxation would work—until we tried them. In fact, we found that the techniques in this section can be transformative as well as comforting, especially while you're coping with chronic illness and pain. The more you practice them, the better you will get at performing them and the more helpful and gratifying they will become.

Self-Hypnosis

If you are able to "see" pictures with your eyes closed, you can hypnotize yourself. All it takes is some simple instruction and practice. With the help of a book, audio recording, or professional hypnotherapist (see Resources), you can learn basic techniques for inducing a state of deep relaxation, such as imagining walking down a staircase as you count backward from ten to one while breathing deeply. Once relaxed, you vividly imagine being in a place—real or imagined—that you find safe and comforting. With this sense of freedom, you can play with ideas pertaining to a specific problem or situation.

You can experiment, for example, with different ways of seeing and coping with your pain. You can be as creative, outlandish, and crazy as you want, because your ideas are only imaginary and only known to you. If you have trouble thinking outside the box, guided visualization recordings are available to provide novel imagery. Amazingly, unexpected and effective ideas may very well pop up when you use visualization in this way. Developing new intervening images can change your behavior and perceptions, augment your concentration and creativity, help you control negative emotions, and build self-esteem.

Meditation

Meditation means different things to different people. Some see it as a form of relaxation, and others use it to access their innate creativity, achieve self-discovery, or acquire spiritual serenity. For everyone, though, meditation connotes "being in the moment," that is, concentrating on your breathing and letting thoughts that so often clutter the mind drift away, leading to a state of calm. While in this state, you can mobilize your deep psychological resources to approach problems with greater concentration and, often, clarity.

If you are new to meditation, you have many options for learning the basic techniques. For example, you can use a book, audio recording, or DVD, or private or classroom instruction (see Resources). You won't need special equipment—just a comfortable, quiet space where you won't be interrupted. Meditation is a soothing activity you can do as often as you wish, for as long a session as you wish. As with self-hypnosis, new, unanticipated ideas may reveal themselves to you regarding how to come to terms with or improve your life situation. At the very least, meditation usually helps its practitioners feel relaxed and refreshed.

Progressive Muscle Relaxation

Progressive muscle relaxation (PMR) is a form of guided imagery that can help you decrease your pain level, increase your ability to relax, and increase your energy and enthusiasm for life. This technique dates back to the 1930s but only came into fashion in the 1980s. Today, many hospitals, libraries, and community education centers offer PMR workshops.

You can learn PMR from a book or by listening to an audio recording (see Resources). There are many variations, but all entail relaxing your muscles through a two-step process. First you deliberately tense certain muscle groups, and then you stop the tension and turn your attention toward how the muscles relax as you release the tension.

With practice you will learn to recognize and distinguish the sensations associated with a tensed muscle and a completely relaxed muscle. With this simple knowledge, you can induce muscular relaxation at the first signs of the tension that accompanies anxiety in your daily life—and inducing physical relaxation reminds you to relax your mind, as well.

Yoga

Developed in India an estimated five thousand years ago, yoga began as a spiritual practice. The original Yogis, practitioners of the ancient Vedic religion, believed that happiness and liberation from earthly suffering arises from union with a divine consciousness. The various yoga practices represent ways of achieving the goal of transcending the self. These days, studies continue to reveal the many health benefits of yoga, making it one of the most popular fitness regimens for workout enthusiasts.

On some level, yoga can be considered a combination of the practice of meditation and stretching exercises. Careful attention to rhythmic breathing directs your thoughts inward, helping you to focus on both the movement of the body and the fluctuations of the mind. Through this process, you come to know your thought patterns without labeling, judging, or trying to change them. In turn, you learn compassion, which can then be directed outward beyond yourself toward the world.

Many people with back problems have found yoga very helpful for their chronic pain. Yoga relaxes and strengthens weak and disfigured spinal muscles and so can be particularly beneficial for those whose muscles have tightened in their attempt to support an uneven spine. But many poses remain off-limits to those with spinal fusions and degenerative disk disease because they call for twisting and arching the back beyond what fragile spines can tolerate.

However, two instructors have developed specialized yoga programs for those with scoliosis. Elise Browning Miller, in California, offers instruction in yoga exercises designed for presurgical scoliosis patients. Ellen Kiley teaches classes and workshops in Maine, Georgia, and throughout the US for postfusion patients, emphasizing certain postures that provide immediate pain relief as well as long-term muscle strengthening and realigning exercises. Over time, these improve body symmetry, increase breathing capacity, and—in Kiley's words—help back pain sufferers "feel powerful, graceful, and whole." See Resources for information about these special programs.

Getting Started

In this chapter, we'll take a look at what it means to learn Pilates. We'll also discuss finding and working with a good instructor. Finally, we'll take a look at several key concepts you'll need to understand before you begin the Pilates exercises.

What Is Pilates?

So, what exactly do people do when they "do Pilates"? There is no standard answer to that question, because unlike many other exercise routines, Pilates programs are highly individualized. That is, Pilates instructors are trained to adapt a series of basic, intermediate, and advanced task-specific exercises to the different physical strengths and limitations of each student.

Generally speaking, though, Pilates workouts take place on floor mats or specially designed equipment. The main piece of equipment, the Universal Reformer, consists of a frame with a padded carriage that slides back and forth within the frame. Adjustable springs attach the carriage to the frame, and the tension can be adjusted with these springs, making it easier or harder to pull or push the carriage along the frame. Other major pieces of equipment include the Trapeze Table (also called the Cadillac) and Wunda Chair.

This equipment provides a means of working on a weak part of the body without putting too much strain on it. For example, if you have had a back injury or surgery that causes pain when you sit or stand, the Pilates equipment places you in a position that reduces the pull of gravity on the fragile section of the spine, thus lessening the chances of activating or exacerbating your pain. You learn to use your abdominal muscles in this position to stabilize your spine, so that when you are once again upright, you will know how to move without re-creating the injury.

As a Pilates student, you progress from highly assisted exercises to more challenging ones that continue to increase in pace and build power, coordination, and flexibility. These exercises all take place on the same apparatuses, with levers, springs, and props adjusted to alter the level of support provided by the machine. During this process, a kind of muscle reeducation takes place. With your new sense of *proprioception,* or awareness of how to move your body through space, you are able to identify and correct problematic movement patterns.

How to Choose an Instructor

To find a trustworthy instructor, we suggest you search the database of the Pilates Method Alliance, an international, not-for-profit professional association dedicated to the teachings of Joseph and Clara Pilates (see Resources). This is a good place to start if no one you know can recommend a favorite instructor.

Once you have identified Pilates instructors in or near your community, you might want to ask the following questions, as suggested by the Pilates Method Alliance:

- Did the instructor attend a comprehensive training program (for example, Power Pilates, Pilates Institute, Polestar Education, Stott, or Body Control Pilates)?

- Did that program require written and practical tests, lectures, observation, and practice and apprentice hours?

- How long has the instructor been teaching Pilates?

- Does the instructor teach the full repertoire of Pilates exercises on all or many of the Pilates equipment?

- Does the instructor have experience with special needs and rehabilitation?

Your instructor should evaluate your needs by observing your postural alignment and having you do some basic exercises while she carefully watches your movement patterns. In this way, she can assess your current range of motion and note any limitations due to weak or imbalanced muscles.

Most likely, you will naturally tend to perform the exercises with your bigger muscles—the hip flexors and rectus abdominus, for example—because they are easier to engage. During your sessions, a good instructor will give verbal, visual, and tactile cues to help you access your deeper muscles.

Over time, you should see your technique improve as your instructor gives you more and more specific cues and you become increasingly familiar with the components of each exercise. In other words, in the beginning, your instructor should allow you to go through the motions so that you simply get a feeling for the gestalt of each exercise. But gradually, she ought to point out how to perform the exercises more precisely using imagery and verbal prompts; for example, she may encourage you to keep some body parts "quiet" or to tense up a muscle so that it is "like steel." As you become proficient, your instructor will taper off the amount of her feedback so that you can begin to rely on internal representations and your own sensory awareness.

Key Concepts

In order to perform Pilates exercises correctly, you must understand and use the following techniques for breathing, spinal positioning, and muscle positioning and movement. It's not enough to do the exercises any old way; they must be combined with these key concepts in order to be effective and safe.

The Breath

Joseph Pilates was asthmatic as a child and lived through the great influenza epidemic of World War I. Consequently, he developed strong opinions about the importance of proper breathing. He came to believe, for example, that the bottom of the lungs was a repository for infection, germs, and disease. Only by fully exhaling could you cleanse the lungs of these toxins, and in order to do so, you had to fully and forcefully push out each exhalation.

In his book, Pilates wrote

To breathe correctly you must completely exhale and inhale, always trying very hard to 'squeeze' every atom of impure air from your lungs in much the same manner that you would wring every drop of water from a wet cloth.... This in turn supplies the bloodstream with vitally necessary life-giving oxygen. Also, the complete exhalation and inhalation of air stimulates all muscles into greater activity. (Pilates and Miller 1998, 13)

The success of a Pilates workout rests on your ability to learn and use a variation of diaphragmatic, or belly, breathing. Belly breathing is the kind of breathing we do naturally when we sleep because it relaxes us, and athletes typically employ it because it is the most efficient way to take in oxygen and get rid of carbon dioxide, a waste product in the body, leading to an increase in energy.

Like belly breathing, Pilates breathing is very different from thoracic breathing, in which you pull a breath of air into your upper torso and shoulders. This action results in a shallow—and not very satisfying or invigorating—breath. If your shoulders and chest are rising to the ceiling, or your upper torso is stiffening up when you inhale, you know you are not breathing correctly.

For correct Pilates breathing, as you inhale, imagine the air is flowing into your sides (and back) and that they are expanding. In this way, you are taking a breath and pushing it to the *sides of your torso*, like a bellows. To make sure you're doing so, when you rest the palms of your hands on the sides of your rib cage, you should be able to feel the area expand outward.

It will probably take a while to figure out how to breathe the Pilates way. With practice, you'll undoubtedly get better at it. But, in the meantime, the most important point to remember is to breathe while you exercise; don't hold your breath.

The Powerhouse

The *powerhouse* is essentially the body's center of gravity. It comprises the muscles of the trunk, including the lower abdomen, lower back, buttocks, and pelvic floor. Engaging the powerhouse during exercise strengthens the transversus abdominis, the deepest layer of abdominal muscles that wrap horizontally around the trunk. By doing so, you develop a strong, corsetlike support system that protects your back from injury.

To feel your powerhouse work, stand up and place one hand on your lower abdomen and the other on your lower back. Inhale deeply through your nose, and then exhale thoroughly through your mouth while pulling the lower abdominals up and toward the spine, simultaneously drawing your pelvic muscles up and squeezing your buttocks together.

Neutral Pelvis

The *neutral pelvis* is another key concept. In order to activate a neutral pelvis, it helps to visualize your skeleton and focus on your pelvis. Lie on your back with your knees bent and your feet flat on the floor. Draw an imaginary line from one hip bone to the other, and two lines down from each hip that meet at your pubic bone, forming a triangle. If you can balance an imaginary cup of coffee on this triangle—because you've tightened it and tilted it slightly upward so that it becomes flat like a small tray—then you've achieved a neutral pelvis.

Navel to Spine

Many people have trouble figuring out how to pull the navel to the spine. To help you understand how it feels to do this, think of how you suck in your belly when you zip up a tight pair of pants. Or, try kneeling in front of a large fitness ball and lean over it with your stomach on the ball. Roll forward just enough so that your hands rest on the floor. Your knees may or may not be off the floor, depending on your size and proportions.

Rest your cheek on the ball and take five breaths, then turn your head and rest the other cheek on the ball for five breaths. Your goal is to inhale deeply without pushing your abdomen into the ball. This action will make your breath expand into the sides and back of your rib cage. As you exhale, pull the belly further up and into the rib cage. Your instructor may remind you to breathe this way by telling you to "scoop" your abdominals or to "knit your ribs together."

At first, you may feel tightness in your back and shoulders, but this will improve as you practice. You might also feel that you can't get a full breath. That's okay. Keep practicing, and eventually this "scooping" or "knitting" of the abdominal muscles will begin to feel more natural and comfortable.

In general, give yourself a couple of months to learn and refine these essential techniques. Slow down your routine so that you can take inventory of your positioning and movements. Observe what you are doing correctly and incorrectly, and strive to improve any problems you notice. Pilates is most effective when you perform it precisely. You're after quality, not quantity or speed.

4

Warm-Up & Mat Exercises
for Fragile Backs

Though Joseph Pilates devised many exercises, we include in this book only those suitable for beginners with spine ailments. It may take you a while to get the positions right, but even as you practice, you will derive a huge benefit as long as you concentrate on moving slowly and as precisely as possible. Remember, precision and control is the goal, because that is what will ultimately enable you to optimize your muscle flexibility and avoid strain and injury.

We insist that you obtain permission from the surgeon who performed your fusion or other surgical procedure, or another medical care provider who fully knows your condition, before beginning any new exercise regimen, including Pilates. For example, you must be sure your bones have fused, within a year or two following fusion surgery, so that the structure of your realigned vertebrae is not compromised.

Also, we strongly encourage you to consult a certified instructor in your community, so the instructor can evaluate your unique needs and so you can be certain that you have mastered the fundamental Pilates positions and techniques before practicing on your own.

The exercises in this chapter have been designed to be performed on a mat. We have modified those exercises for fragile backs. You should concentrate on the mat exercises, since these will be the ones you can do both in a studio with an instructor and at home by yourself. In chapters 5 and 6, we'll discuss exercises on Pilates equipment (the Reformer and the Cadillac).

Pre-Pilates Warm-Up Exercises

These exercises warm up the muscles in the shoulders, head, neck, spine, and legs. As well, they correctly position the body for the rest of the workout. Keep in mind that when practicing Pilates, you concentrate on the powerhouse—roughly the area underneath the chest to the top of the thighs. Once the powerhouse strengthens, you can incorporate a systematic, integrated approach of building the muscles of the extremities.

PRE-PILATES WARM-UP #1

1. Lie on your back with your knees bent, your feet on the mat, and your arms straight by your sides, resting on the mat, and begin to inhale and exhale normally.

2. With pelvis in neutral position, continue breathing, then knit the ribs together by pulling them toward the center of your trunk, and allow your powerhouse to melt into the mat. It's important to keep your back fully pressed into the mat, since it is from this position that the spine corrects itself in reclining exercises.

3. On an inhalation, raise your hands to the ceiling with the palms facing one another; your shoulders should rise off the matt. Drop your shoulders down to the mat on an exhalation, allowing your powerhouse to melt more deeply into the mat.

4. With your hands still raised to the ceiling, turn your palms toward your feet, and inhale. Exhale as you lower your arms to hip level, slightly above the mat.

Repeat five times.

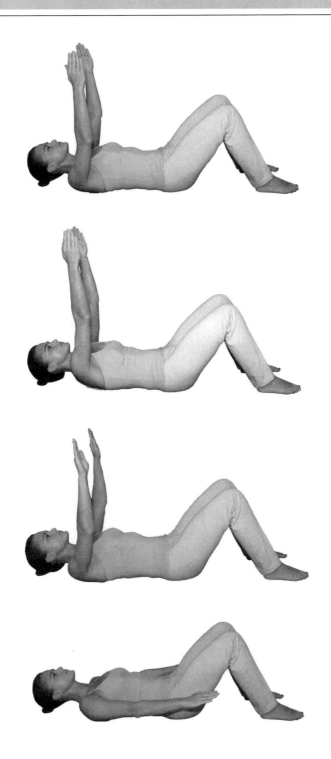

1. With the powerhouse imprinted evenly into the mat, raise both legs into a tabletop position—that is, with your thighs at a ninety-degree angle to the mat (straight up) and your shins parallel to the floor. If one were to set a table for dinner on your shins, nothing should fall off.

2. From this position, slowly drop one foot at a time, with only the big toe touching the mat. Inhale each time you drop your foot, and exhale while raising it. Repeat, alternating feet.

Repeat five times on each foot.

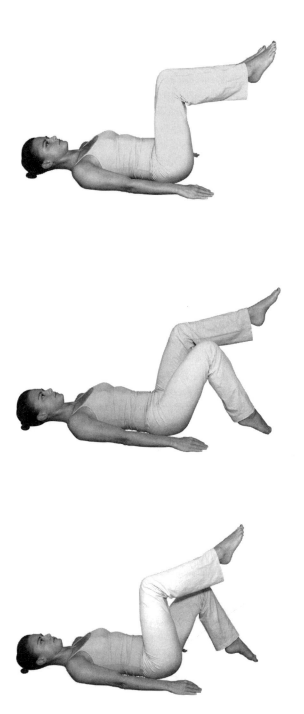

Exercise Routine on the Mat

Here is the Pilates routine on the mat, modified for people with fragile backs

ONE HUNDRED

This exercise is sometimes referred to as "slapping water."

1. Lie on your back with your knees bent and feet on the mat or legs in tabletop position, whichever is more comfortable for you. Support your neck by placing a small, shallow pillow (or folded bath towel) under your head.

2. Keeping your back flat on the mat, extend your arms from the shoulder toward your feet, approximately at the level of your abdomen. Keep your arms straight and your back flat and melted into the mat.

3. Begin to pump your arms up and down, to the sides of and above the abdominal cavity, keeping them long and straight.

4. Pump five times with one deep inhalation and five times with one deep exhalation.

Repeat until you have done one hundred pumps with ten inhalations and exhalations.

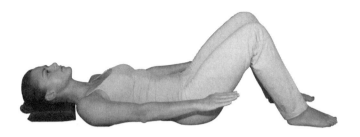

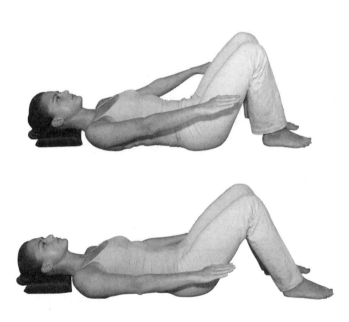

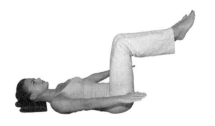

- Advanced "Tabletop"
  Position for One Hundred

HALF ROLL BACK

1. Sit on the mat with your knees bent, kneecaps facing the ceiling, and feet flat on the mat. Hold the backs of your thighs, under the knees, with your hands. Keep your elbows up and out, away from the powerhouse. Knit your ribs together, scooping your abdomen.

2. On an inhale breath, begin by slowly rolling the base of the spine down toward the mat as you scoop, scoop, scoop. Continue rolling back, bone by bone, while walking the hands down the backs of the thighs for support. Continue to the point where your feet are just about to come up off the mat. If your feet come up off the mat, you've gone back too far.

3. As you exhale, maintaining your scooped abdomen or C-curve, slowly come back to your original, seated position, vertebra by vertebra, while walking your hands back up to your knees.

Repeat five times.

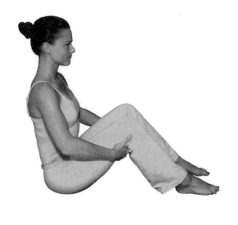

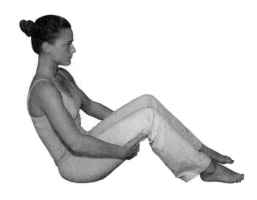

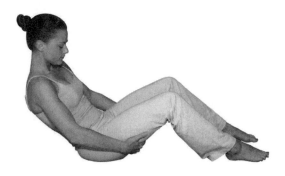

SINGLE LEG CIRCLES

1. Lie flat on the mat, with your head on a pillow or folded towel. Bend one leg, kneecap facing the ceiling and foot on the mat. Your arms should be straight at your sides and flat on the mat.

2. Bring the other knee to your chest and straighten that leg toward the ceiling. With your powerhouse pressed into the mat, begin to draw small, imaginary circles on the ceiling with the toe of the extended foot. Make sure your raised leg slightly crosses the inner thigh of the bent leg.

3. It is imperative that your hips remain stable. If your hips rock, draw smaller circles.

4. Repeat five times, then reverse direction (in other words, if you started by circling to the left, now circle to the right). Switch to the other leg and repeat five times in each direction.

Repeat the entire exercise five times.

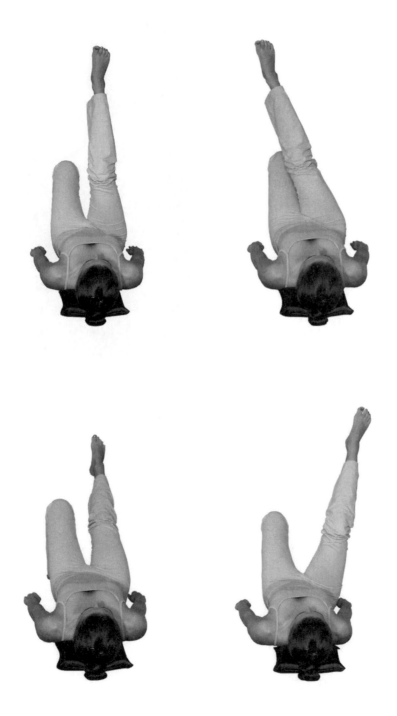

SINGLE LEG STRETCH

1. Lie on your back with both legs extended at a ninety-degree angle to the mat (straight up) and a pillow or towel beneath your head. Your pelvis should be in a neutral position, and your back should be flat against the mat. Lightly hold on to one knee with both hands. Keep your elbows open and lifted so that your abs and legs, rather than your arms, are doing the work.

2. On an inhale breath, knit the ribs together (pull your navel to your spine) and bend the knee you are holding in to your chest while the other knee remains at a ninety-degree angle to the mat. Keep the back of your neck relaxed and long.

3. Exhale while switching legs.

Repeat five times.

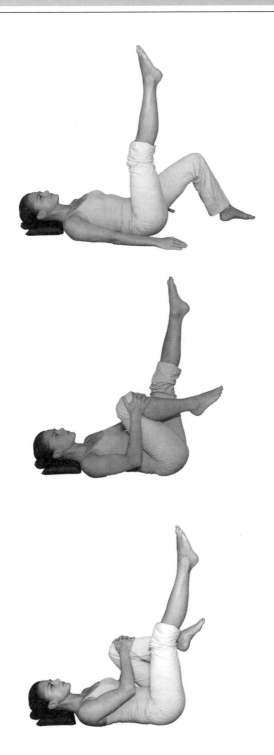

DOUBLE LEG STRETCH

1. Lie on your back with your legs at a
    ninety-degree angle to the mat (straight
    up) and a pillow or towel beneath your
    head. Inhale deeply and knit your ribs
    together (pull your navel to your spine, or
    scoop, scoop, scoop!).

2. Extend your arms straight up and slightly
    back. As you exhale, circle your arms
    around (as if you're about to hug a big
    ball) and then toward your feet. Pull your
    knees in to your chest, grabbing your
    ankles or whatever you can comfortably
    reach.

3. Return your legs to a ninety-degree angle. If you
    feel ready to advance to a more challenging
    version of this exercise, you can put your legs in
    tabletop position instead of at ninety degrees to
    the mat.

Repeat five times.

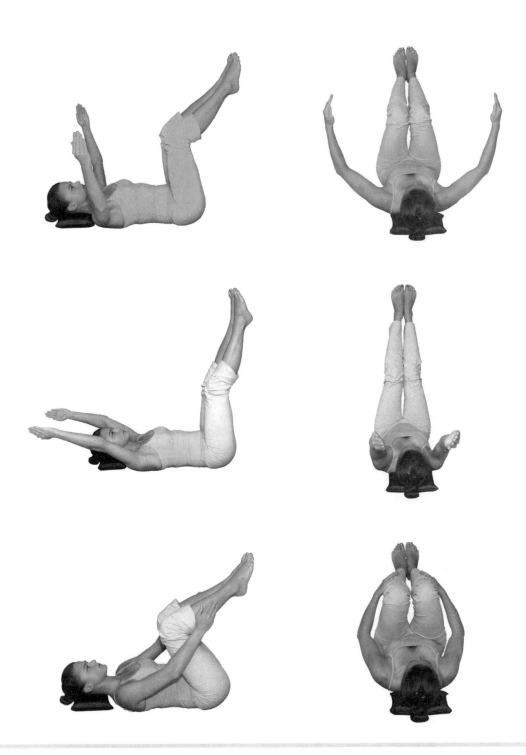

SCISSORS

1. Lie on your back with both legs at a ninety-degree angle to the mat (straight up) and a pillow or towel beneath your head. If this is too strenuous, leave one leg bent, kneecap facing the ceiling and foot flat on the floor.

2. Inhale. Lift one leg straight up to the ceiling. As you exhale, raise your arms with elbows wide and lightly hold on to the elevated leg, wherever you can comfortably reach. Pulse that leg twice toward your chest. Exhale as you switch legs. In the event that you have any pain, keep the extended leg slightly bent.

Repeat five times.

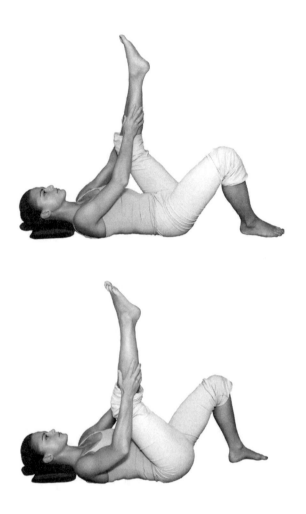

LOWER LEGS LIFT

1. Lie on your back with both legs slightly bent, raised and pointed toward the ceiling, or in tabletop position. Place a pillow or towel beneath your head. Place your hands underneath the "sitting" bones in your buttocks. With your back pressed into the mat, knit your ribs together.

2. While inhaling, lower both legs slightly, about three inches, and follow with an exhale breath as you return your legs to their original position. The range of movement here should be quite limited.

Repeat five times.

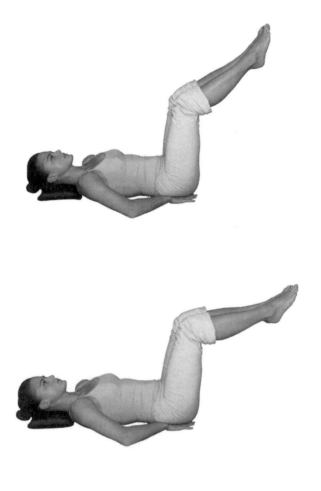

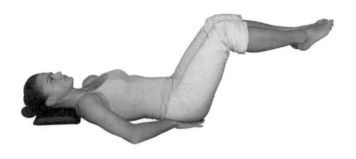

SPINE STRETCH FORWARD

1. Sit tall with your feet mat width apart, shoulders directly over the hips, feet flexed, and both legs pushed into the mat or slightly bent, whichever is more comfortable for you. Stretch both arms straight out in front of you at shoulder height. Inhale.

2. On an exhale breath, leading with your head, slowly reach your arms toward your feet. Allow your back to form a shallow C. As you continue to lean forward, the C-curve should increase, as should the stretch through the spine. Continue to reach your hands toward your feet. Keep your hips stable.

3. As you inhale, slowly return, vertebra by vertebra, to a sitting tall position. Reduce your movement forward if you have any pain or discomfort.

Repeat five times.

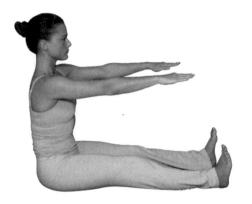

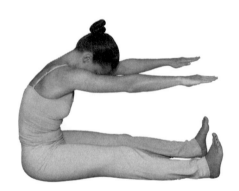

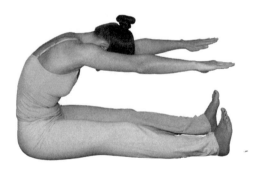

SIDE LEG KICKS

1. Lie on your side, hip stacked on hip, and shoulder on shoulder. You may hold your head up with your bent elbow or lay the side of your head on your outstretched arm on the mat. The entire side of your body should be aligned and straight. Flex your feet to elongate the legs. Your tailbone should be tucked in, to protect the back. Make sure you pull your abs up and in.

2. As you inhale, slowly lift your top leg about three inches above the mat. Lengthen the top leg forward in front of your body, pulsing it twice toward your head.

3. As you exhale, return your top leg to align with your bottom leg and swing your leg behind you. Return your top leg to align with your bottom leg and lower your raised foot to meet your other foot. Keep your hips aligned. If you find you cannot, reduce your range of motion (that is, don't kick so far forward or behind you).

Repeat five times on each side.

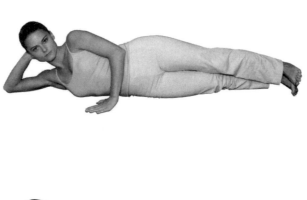

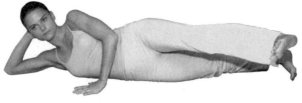

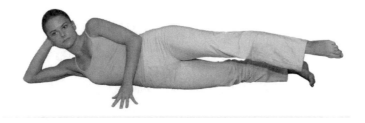

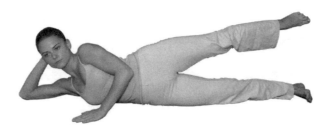

POSTMAT COOLDOWN: THE WALL

1. With your heels touching and your feet forming a V, stand approximately one foot away from a wall and rest your back against it. Gently push your entire spine against the wall, making sure each vertebra, as well as your waist and shoulders, is firmly pressed into the wall. Sink your ribs into the wall so there's no space between you and the wall.

2. With your abs up and in, begin to peel yourself off the wall, starting with your head, as though you were being torn off of a piece of Velcro. Continue with your shoulders, and then one vertebra after the other, until your head is bending over and your hands are hanging loosely at your knees. As you roll down, pull the abs in more deeply.

3. With your arms hanging lazily toward the floor, slowly circle them toward one another, swinging from the shoulder, five times. Reverse direction and circle another five times. Slowly, with control, roll the spine, waist, and head back to the wall, bone by bone. If your fusion prohibits bending at the waist or hips, you can remain flush with the wall.

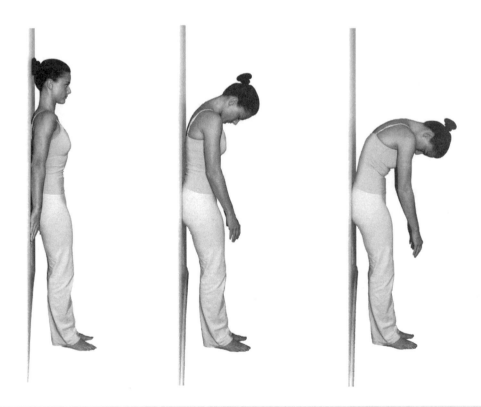

5

Reformer Exercises for Fragile Backs

Once you have mastered the mat exercises, your instructor may want to vary your workout by adding exercises on the Reformer and the Cadillac. Please work individually with a Pilates instructor as you learn these exercises. In the future, you might prefer to join a group class or purchase your own Reformer, but do so only when you and your instructor agree that you have mastered this workout.

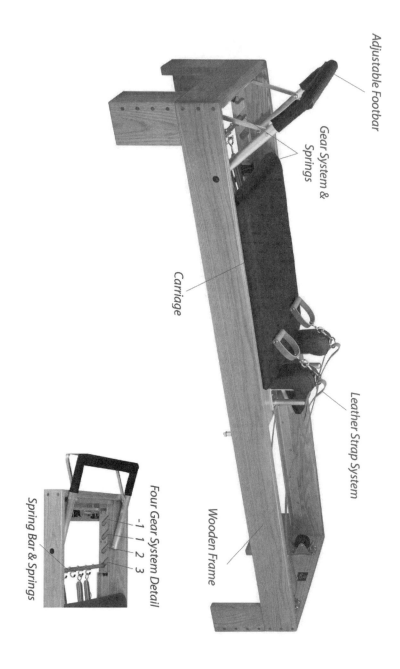

Adjustable Footbar

Gear System & Springs

Carriage

Leather Strap System

Wooden Frame

Four Gear System Detail

-1 1 2 3

Spring Bar & Springs

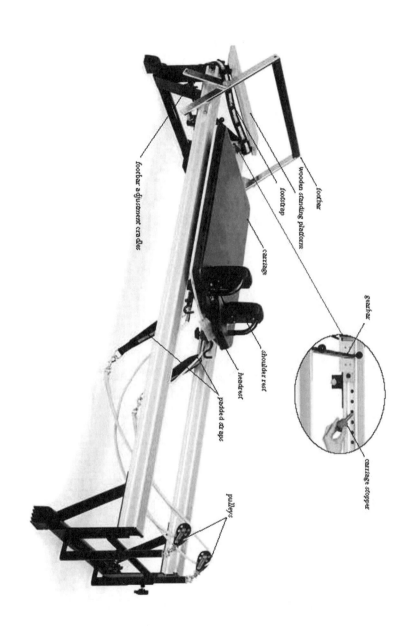

footbar adjustment cradles

wooden standing platform

footbar

footstrap

carriage

gearbar

shoulder rest

headrest

padded straps

carriage stopper

pulleys

TOES

1. Starting with light springs (2 to 2½
    instead of 3½ to 4), lie on your back with
    a pillow or towel beneath your head on
    the headrest. Place your toes on the foot
    bar with your heels together, forming a **V**.
    Exhale.

2. As you inhale, with your abs pulled up
    and in, push away from the bar. Fully
    extend your legs. Then bend your knees,
    exhale, and return, with control, to the
    bar. Repeat five times slowly and with
    precision.

3. Do another five repetitions, finding a nice
    rhythm and flow through the movements.

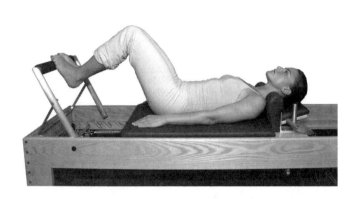

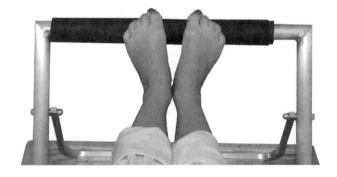

ARCHES

1. Continue the footwork exercises by placing the arches of each foot on the foot bar, with your toes long and your heels around the bar, like a bird on a perch. Your feet should be parallel to one another.

2. As you inhale, with your abs pulled up and in, push away from the bar. Fully extend your legs, keeping your knees together, and pause briefly while pushing your heels down. Then bend your knees, exhale, and return—with control—to the bar. Repeat five times slowly and with precision.

3. For the second five repetitions, find a nice rhythm and flow through the movements.

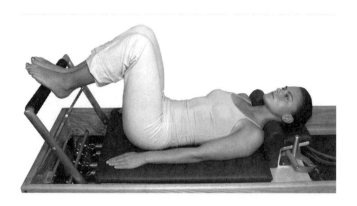

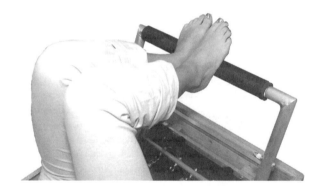

HEELS

1. Continue the footwork exercises by placing your heels on the foot bar with your ankles flexed, toes back toward your head. Your feet should be parallel to one another.

2. As you inhale, with your abs pulled up and in, push away from the bar. Fully extend your legs, keeping your knees together and continuing to flex your ankles. Then bend the knees, exhale, and return—with control—to the bar. Repeat five times slowly and with precision.

3. For the second five repetitions, find a nice rhythm and flow through the movements.

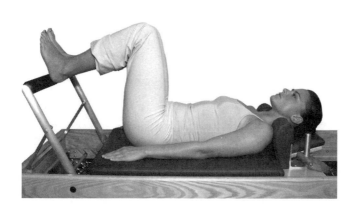

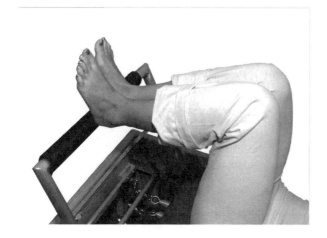

TENDON STRETCH

1. Continue the footwork exercises by placing the toes of both feet on the foot bar, with your toes apart and heels high and together (as if you are on tiptoe).

2. With your abs pulled up and in, inhale, and push away from the bar. Fully extend your legs, keeping your knees together. With your legs straight, exhale and drop only the heels, then lift your feet back into tiptoe position. Repeat five times slowly and with precision.

3. For the second five repetitions, find a nice rhythm and flow through the movements.

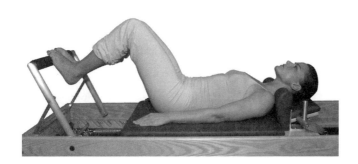

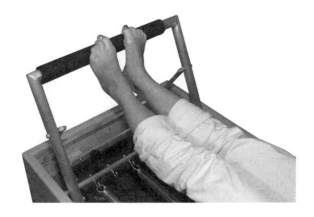

ONE HUNDRED

1. Starting with light springs (2 to 2½ instead of 3½ to 4), lie on your back with a pillow or towel beneath your head on the headrest. Hold the handles like mittens and extend your arms straight toward your feet. Keep your hands flat, your fingers together, and your palms down. Put your legs in tabletop position or, if it is more comfortable, with your knees to your chest.

2. Pump your arms toward your feet, on either side of and above the abdomen, five times to each inhale and five to each exhale, holding your arms stiffly from the back of the shoulders.

Repeat until you have done one hundred pumps with ten inhalations and exhalations.

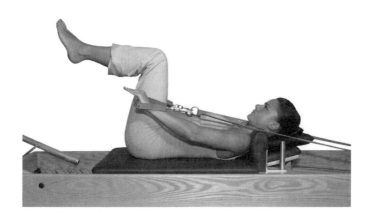

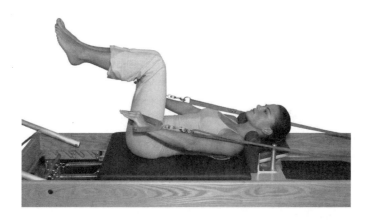

FROG LEGS

1. Add an extension strap to your handles. Starting with very light springs (1½), lie on your back with a pillow or towel beneath your head on the headrest. Pull one foot to your chest, and place a loop over the arch of that foot while pushing the carriage back with the other. Pull your other foot to your chest and slip a loop over that foot, as well. (Your instructor will help you learn this maneuver.) Rest your tailbone on the mat with your knees wide apart and your heels pulled in toward your tailbone.

2. Inhale deeply and extend your legs straight out toward the foot bar and on a high diagonal. Exhale, and slowly, with control, return to your original position with your knees splayed, like a frog. If this movement causes discomfort, you can keep your legs at a ninety-degree angle to the carriage (straight up).

Repeat five times.

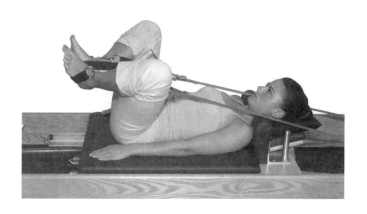

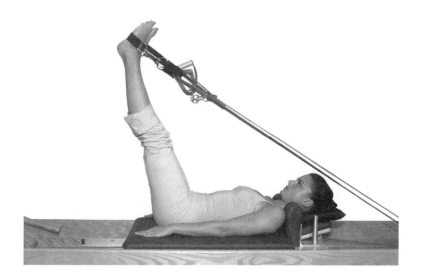

LEG CIRCLES

1. With the extension straps still around your feet, extend your legs straight at a ninety-degree angle to the carriage (straight up).

2. Keeping your feet parallel and together, lower your legs to a forty-five degree angle. Separate your legs and swing the right leg to the right and then up, while swinging the left leg to the left and then up. Both feet should meet at the ninety-degree angle position. Slowly draw five imaginary circles with each leg in this way.

3. Reverse the direction and draw five more circles. As you get stronger, you may be able to lower your legs closer to the mat.

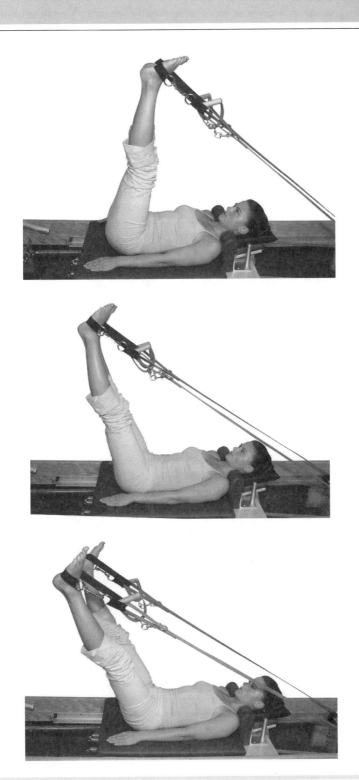

ROUND BACK STOMACH MASSAGE

To the instructor: *Avoid teaching the round back stomach massage if the location of the fusion or injury prevents your client from getting into position. Over time, as the client's powerhouse gets stronger, you can introduce this exercise.*

1. Starting with moderate springs (2½), sit tall in the front and center of the carriage. Place both feet on the foot bar, toes apart, heels together and raised, forming a V. With bent knees, hold on to the front end of the carriage with each hand—your left hand to the left of your left foot, and your right hand to the right of your right foot—keeping your elbows up and wide.

2. Inhale. Extend your legs long and straight. With straight legs, drop and lift your heels once. As you exhale, bend your knees and elbows. Leading with the pelvis, scoop to return.

Repeat four to five times.

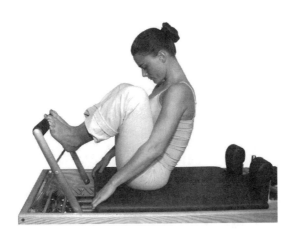

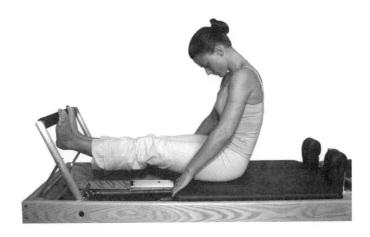

STRAIGHT BACK STOMACH MASSAGE

1. Remain on the carriage, sitting tall with your feet on the foot bar in a V. Your knees should be bent. Wrap each hand around each shoulder rest behind you and straighten your arms.

2. Inhale. Extend your legs long and straight. With straight legs, drop and lift your heels once. As you exhale, bend your knees to return to the foot bar.

Repeat four to five times.

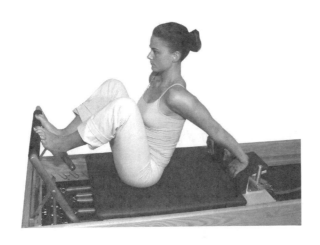

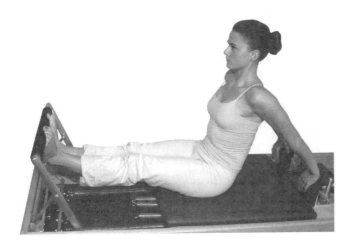

ELEPHANT

To the instructor: *Even clients with rod and pedicle fusions can perform this exercise and benefit greatly from it. The powerhouse is heavily involved, so a client's inflexibility does not prevent proper positioning and movement.*

1. Use 2 springs. Facing the foot bar, carefully mount the carriage by placing your near hand on the foot bar and your far leg on the carriage with your foot against the far shoulder rest. Repeat using your far hand and near foot. Both hands should be holding on to the foot bar, and both feet should be against the shoulder rests. Point your toes to the ceiling.

2. Lower your head so you are looking into the carriage. Scoop your abs while "doming" your back. Round up from the pelvis to the breastbone, and begin to push your legs and the carriage backward. Keep your toes pointed upward and your heels flat on the carriage.

3. Return by bringing your tailbone under you as you deepen the powerhouse. The carriage will be dragged back to the foot bar as you pull your abs up and in. Keep your upper body quiet and your shoulders down and relaxed throughout this exercise.

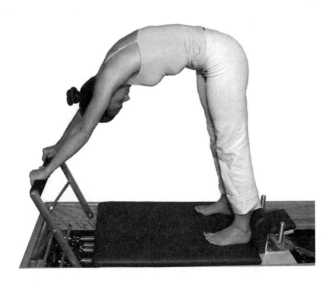

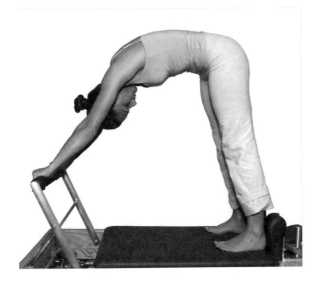

KNEE STRETCH (ROUND BACK)

1. Starting with 2 springs, carefully mount the carriage by placing your near hand on the foot bar and your far knee on the carriage with your foot against the far shoulder rest. Repeat using your far hand and near knee and foot. Straighten your arms, scoop your abs, and tuck your tailbone under you.

2. Inhale as you sit back close to your heels, then push your knees out behind you—only for a very short distance, the length of your shins. Keep the upper body quiet and stable.

3. Exhale as you return by deepening the powerhouse, resisting the springs and maintaining control as you drag the carriage back to the foot bar. Your thighs should remain disengaged in this exercise; the powerhouse should be doing all the work.

Repeat five times.

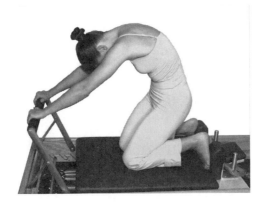

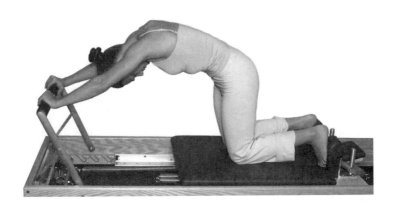

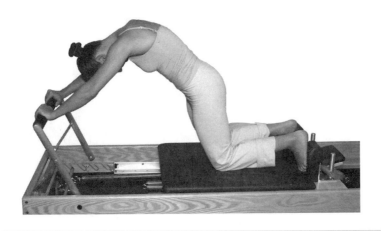

Reformer Exercises for Fragile Backs   125

RUNNING

1. Starting with 2½ to 3 springs, lie on your back with a pillow or towel beneath your head on the headrest. Place your toes on the foot bar with feet parallel to one another.

2. Lower one heel while bending the knee of the opposite leg. Prance in this way with control. Keep the hips stable and completely still throughout the exercise. Focus on your toes as they push up and down, away from the foot bar.

Repeat twenty times.

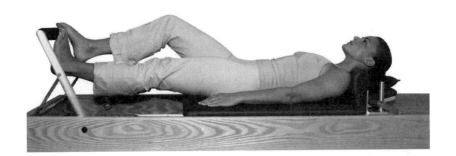

PELVIC LIFT

1. Starting with 2½ to 3 springs, lie on your back with a pillow or towel beneath your head on the headrest. Place the arches of each foot on the farthest corners of the foot bar. Lift your pelvis up off the carriage while leaving the last rib down on the carriage. Inhale and extend your legs long and straight, keeping your pelvis above the carriage.

2. On an exhale breath, slowly return by dragging the "sitting" bones in your buttocks back to the foot bar.

Repeat six to ten times.

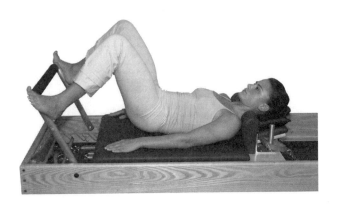

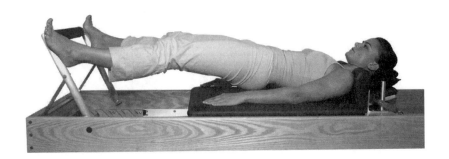

Cadillac Exercises for Fragile Backs

We recommend that you work with a Pilates instructor as you learn these exercises. In the future, you might prefer to join a class or purchase your own Cadillac, but do so only when you and your instructor agree that you have mastered these exercises.

Peak Cadillac

Roll Down Bar
& Leg Springs

Hanging Straps

Table Mat

Trapeze & Precision Slider

Push-Through
Bar

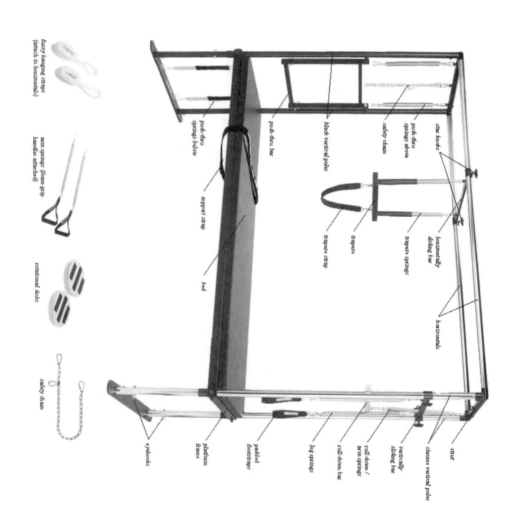

fuzzy hanging straps
(attach to horizontal)

arm springs (foam-grip
handles attached)

rotational disks

safety chain

push-thru
springs below

push-thru
springs above

push-thru bar

black vertical pole

safety chain

star knobs

support strap

trapeze strap

trapeze

trapeze springs

horizontally
sliding bar

bed

horizontal

eyehooks

platform
frame

padded
footstraps

leg springs

roll-down bar

roll-down /
arm springs

vertically
sliding bar

chrome vertical pole

strut

If you have muscle stiffness in your back, keep your knees bent for this exercise.

1. Facing the roll-down bar and with your knees slightly bent, place the soles of your feet on the base of the perpendicular poles of the Cadillac. Place both hands on the bar, thumbs joining the fingers around the bar, shoulder width apart. Inhale.

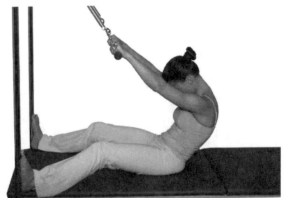

2. As you exhale, slowly begin to roll down, vertebra by vertebra, toward the mat of the Cadillac. Control the speed of the roll by knitting your ribs and deepening the **C**-curve of the powerhouse. Make sure the roll-down bar is even throughout this series of movements. Inhale.

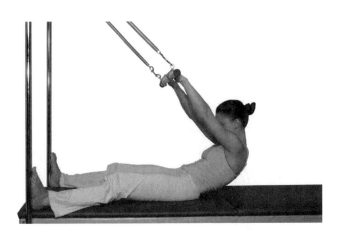

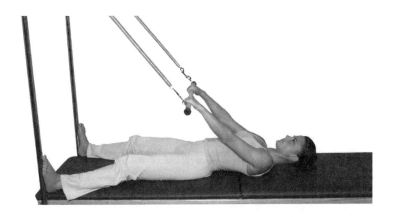

3. Exhale deeply and return by peeling your
   spine off the mat, vertebra by vertebra,
   deepening the powerhouse as you come
   back to a seated position.

Repeat three times.

BREATHING A (PULL-DOWN)

1. Lie on your back so that your head is under the roll-down bar, a hand's distance away from the edge of the Cadillac.

2. Place both feet in the trapeze while holding on to the roll-down bar, above you, with both hands, thumbs joining the fingers around the bar. With straight arms, inhale, push the bar down to your hips, and hold your breath for a count of three.

3. Exhale, and return the bar, with control, to your starting position.

Repeat three times.

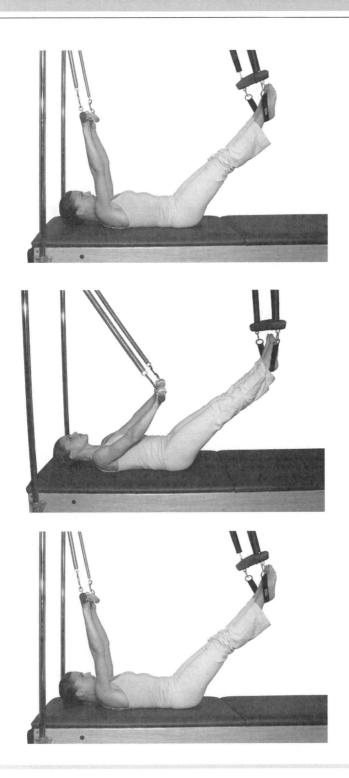

BREATHING B (PELVIC LIFT)

1. Lie on your back. You should still be holding the roll-down bar with both hands, thumbs joining the fingers around the bar. Inhale and knit the ribs together (pull your navel to your spine, or scoop, scoop, scoop).

2. With your arms quiet and your feet in the trapeze, lift your pelvis off the Cadillac. Hold your breath for a count of three. Exhale, and with control, return your pelvis to the Cadillac.

Repeat three times.

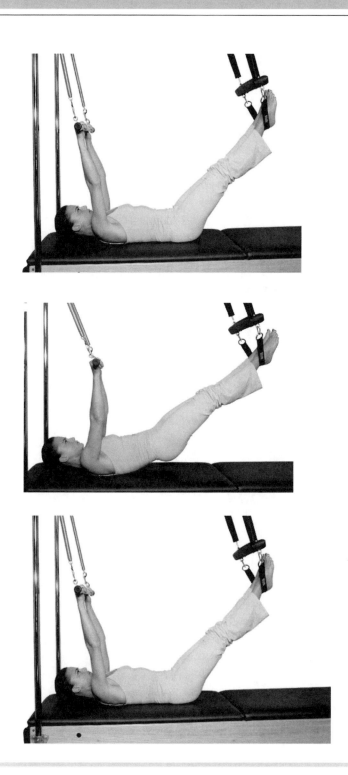

BREATHING C (PULL-DOWN & PELVIC LIFT)

1. Lie on your back. For this exercise, simultaneously push the roll-down bar down and lift your pelvis up off the mat. Hold your breath for a count of three.

2. Exhale, and with control, simultaneously return your pelvis to the Cadillac and return the roll-down bar to your starting position. If you have any discomfort, bend your knees with feet flat on the Cadillac rather than placing your legs in the trapeze.

Repeat three times.

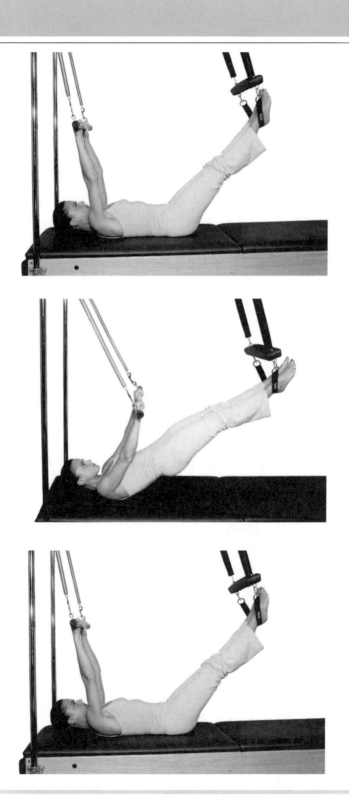

7

Final Thoughts

Joseph Pilates, creator of the Pilates method, once wrote that his exercise regimen "develops the body uniformly, corrects wrong postures, restores physical vitality, invigorates the mind, and elevates the spirit" (Pilates and Miller 1998, 9). His impact on the world of fitness and exercise was nothing short of revolutionary. His original thirty-four exercises and those he developed throughout his career were carefully designed based on decades of scientific study, experimentation, and research into the variety of problems and complications that upset the body's balance and coordination.

The Pilates method has proved to be effective for those who want to maintain a healthy spine. But more importantly, it addresses the problems and limitations associated with spinal disorders. It can be particularly effective for those with fragile spines or spine disorders who would prefer to avoid surgery if at all possible and for some people who are preparing for surgery. And Pilates offers rehabilitation and pain reduction to people who have already undergone spinal surgery, because it strengthens the trunk muscles that support and protect the spine.

However, you must use caution when learning and practicing Pilates, with or without a trainer, and you must maintain a healthy respect for your own physical limits. Go slowly, even though some of the exercises may seem too easy or simple. Keep in mind that when you practice this introductory routine consistently and precisely, it will be far more helpful to your spine than other exercise regimens that involve more repetitions, longer workout sessions, or more vigorous movements. Pilates has proven to be extremely gentle on the joints, yet it is intense and highly effective. Done correctly, Pilates will most likely lead to positive results. You may feel some relief even after the first lesson, but for long-term benefits, your patience and faith are required.

When you realize that other exercise and physical therapy methods don't work, that prescription and nonprescription medications can only do so much (and frequently with uncomfortable side effects), and that new and better pain medications may take a long time to show up at your local pharmacy, it's time to move on to something better. It's time to give Pilates a try.

It may be that you always experience a degree of pain, but it's not necessary for pain to control your life. A safe and effective exercise regimen takes time, effort, and persistence. With Pilates, we have taken back our lives. You can take yours back, too.

Resources

Products

Most of these helpful products can be found online.

Lumbar and Cervical Supports

McKenzie Lumbar Roll (standard or firm), **Cervical Roll, Night Roll, Super and D-Section Rolls with elastic straps**
    Available at any online medical devices purveyor and at medical supply stores.

Adjustable Firmness Mattresses

Sleep Number Beds
    Available at www.selectcomfort.com or any Select Comfort store.

TENS Units

Intelect Standard TENS Unit (#77687)

Available at any online medical devices purveyor and at medical supply stores.

DVDs, Workshops, Retreats, and Books

Yoga for Scoliosis

DVD, books, and workshops by Elise Browning Miller.

Available at www.yogaforscoliosis.com.

Relaxation Body Scan and Guided Imagery for Well-Being

Progressive muscle relaxation audio CD by Carolyn McManus.

Available at www.amazon.com.

Mindfulness Meditation: Cultivating the Wisdom of Your Body and Mind

Meditation audio CD by Jon Kabat-Zinn.

Available at www.amazon.com.

Self-Hypnosis

Audio recording by Matthew McKay.

Available at www.newharbinger.com.

Scoliyogi

Yoga retreats in Maine, Georgia, and throughout the US for postsurgical scoliosis patients by Ellen Kiley.

www.scoliyogi.com

Organizations

National Scoliosis Foundation

Provides a periodic publication, *The Spinal Connection,* and maintains a list of orthopedic specialists, support groups, and other information on scoliosis.

(781) 341-6333 or (800) 673-6922, or www.scoliosis.org

Scoliosis Research Society

Publishes a newsletter, maintains a listing of physicians, and provides information.

(414) 289-9107 or www.srs.org

The National Pain Foundation

An online education and support community for people in pain and their families.

www.nationalpainfoundation.org

Spine Health and Illness Web Sites

www.spine-dr.com (created by a group of spine physicians)

www.spine-health.com

www.spineuniverse.com

www.orthospine.com

Finding Qualified Instructors & Practitioners

Pilates Instructors

Pilates Method Alliance (nonprofit organization)

www.pilatesmethodalliance.org

Power Pilates

www.powerpilates.com

Pilates PhysicalMind Institute

www.themethodpilates.com

Pilates Institute (Texas)

www.pilates-institute.com

Polestar Education

www.polestareducation.com

Pilates Center

www.thepilatescenter.com

Stott Pilates (Canada)

www.stottpilates.com

Body Control Pilates (UK)

www.bodycontrol.co.uk

Psychotherapists &
Chronic Illness Support Groups

National Association of Social Workers (NASW)

www.naswdc.org

Anxiety Disorders Association of America

www.adaa.org (click on Getting Help/Find a Therapist)

Association for Behavioral and Cognitive Therapies

www.abct.org (click on Find a Therapist)

You can also ask your primary medical care provider or health insurance company for a recommendation, or contact the psychiatric outpatient service or mental health department of the closest major hospital.

Massage Therapists

National Certification Board for Therapeutic Massage and Bodywork

www.ncbtmb.com (click on Find Practitioners in Your Area)

Craniosacral Massage Therapists

Upledger Institute

www.upledger.com (click on Find a Practitioner)

Hypnotherapists

National Board for Certified Clinical Hypnotherapists

www.natboard.com

American Society of Clinical Hypnosis

www.asch.net (click on Looking for a Referral?)

Internet Support Forums

Chronic Pain Assistance

for those with chronic pain

http://health.groups.yahoo.com/group/Chronic_Pain_Assistance

National Scoliosis Foundation

for those with scoliosis

http://forums.scoliosis-support.com

FeistyScolioFlatbackers

for those who will need or had a revised fusion procedure

http://health.groups.yahoo.com/group/FeistyScolioFlatbackers

Flatback Revised

for those who will need or had a revised fusion procedure

http://health.groups.yahoo.com/group/Flatback_Revised

Pumpsters

for those who use a morphine pain pump

http://health.groups.yahoo.com/group/pumpsters

References

Ahsan, S. K. 1997. Metabolism of magnesium in health and disease. *Journal of the Indian Medical Association* 95:507–10.

American Academy of Orthopaedic Surgeons. 2000. National ambulatory medical care survey. www.aaos.org.

Anderson, T., F. B. Christensen, E. S. Hansen, and C. Bunger. 2003. Pain five years after instrumented and non-instrumented posterolateral lumbar spinal fusion. *European Spine Journal* 12:393–99.

Brosseau, L., S. Milne, V. Robinson, S. Marchand, B. Shea, G. Wells, and P. Tugwell. 2002. Efficacy of transcutaneous electrical nerve stimulation for the treatment of chronic low back pain: A meta-analysis. *Spine* 27:596–603.

Cherkin, D., D. Eisenberg, K. J. Sherman, W. Barlow, T. J. Kaptchuk, J. Street, and R. A. Deyo. 2001. Randomized trial comparing traditional Chinese medical acupuncture, therapeutic massage, and self-care education for chronic low back pain. *Archives of Internal Medicine* 161:1081–88.

Deyo, R. A. 2004. Spinal-fusion surgery: The case for restraint. *New England Journal of Medicine* 350:722–26.

Foster, L., L. Clapp, M. Erickson, and B. Jabbari. 2001. Botulinum toxin A and chronic low back pain: A randomized, double-blind study. *Neurology* 56:1290–93.

Gunzburg, R., M. Szpalski, and G. B. J. Andersson, eds. 2004. *Degenerative Disc Disease.* Philadelphia: Lippincott Williams & Wilkins.

Healthcare Cost and Utilization Project. 2003. National statistics: Intervertebral disc disorders 2003. www.hcup.ahrq.gov.

Herkowitz, A. J. 1998. Indications for thoracic and lumbar spine fusion and trends in use. *Orthopedic Clinics of North America* 29:803.

Nadler, S. F., D. J. Steiner, G. N. Erasala, D. A. Hengehold, R. T. Hinkle, M. Beth Goodale, S. B. Abeln, and K. W. Weingand. 2002. Continuous low-level heat wrap therapy provides more efficacy than ibuprofen and acetaminophen for acute low back pain. *Spine* 27:1012–17.

Neuwirth, M. 1996. *The Scoliosis Handbook.* New York: Henry Holt and Company.

Pilates, J., and W. J. Miller. 1998. *Return to Life Through Contrology.* Boston: Christopher Publishing House.

Preyde, M. 2000. Effectiveness of massage therapy for subacute low-back pain. *Canadian Medical Association Journal* 162:1815–20.

Urban, J. P. G., and S. Roberts. 2003. Degeneration of the intervertebral disc. *Arthritis Research and Therapy* 5:120–30.

Wilkinson, H. A. 1983. The role of improper surgery in the etiology of the failed back syndrome. In *The Failed Back Syndrome: Etiology and Therapy*. Philadelphia: J. B. Lippincott.

Zeegers, W. S. 1999. Artificial disc replacement with the modular type SB Charité III: Two-year results in fifty prospectively studied patients. *European Spine Journal* 8:210–17.

Andra Fischgrund Stanton, LICSW, an independent, licensed psychiatric social worker, has been practicing individual and marital psychotherapy for twenty-five years, most recently at University of Massachusetts-Memorial Hospital. Over the years she has been especially sensitive to clients with chronic illness as she herself has been coping with scoliosis and back pain since the age of eleven. Currently she writes from her home in Concord, MA.

Certified through the Power Pilates Method in New York City, **Ruth Hiatt-Coblentz** has earned advanced certification in Pilates mat, Reformer, Cadillac and Wunda Chair instruction. She has a degree in History and Near Eastern Studies from Clark University. In her private studio, Think Pilates in Worcester, MA, she finds particular satisfaction helping those with fragile spines, having had three spinal surgeries of her own.

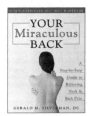
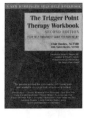
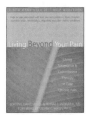
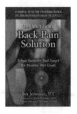
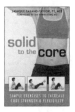